HOW TO BECOME
THE PARENT YOU NEVER HAD

HOW TO BECOME THE PARENT YOU NEVER HAD

A treatment for extremes of Fear, Anger and Guilt

GEOFF GRAHAM B.D.S.

REAL OPTIONS PRESS

First published in Great Britain 1986 by
Real Options Press
Dunsopp House
Lucy Street
Blaydon upon Tyne
NE21 5PU

© Geoff Graham 1986
All rights reserved. No part of this book may be reproduced or transmitted in any form or by any means whatsoever without prior written permission from the publisher except in the case of brief quotations embodied in critical articles and reviews.

British Library Cataloguing in Publication Data
Graham, Geoff
How to become the parent you never had: a treatment for extremes of fear, anger and guilt.
1. Psychotherapy
I. Title
616.89'14   RC480
ISBN 0 9511951 0 7

Printed by Martin's of Berwick, Sea View Works, Spittal, Berwick upon Tweed, TD15 1RS.

Contents

	Page
Introduction	1
Chapter 1.	
The Marathon and The Purpose of Life Itself.	3
Chapter 2.	
Behaviour at Birth—Negative Imprinting.	
—First Line Trauma.	11
Chapter 3.	
From a few hours after birth to six years of age,	
—Negative Imprinting and Conditioning.	
—Second Line Trauma.—Cry for Attention	25
Chapter 4.	
From four years of age to the present day,	
—Negative Conditioning.	
—Third Line Trauma.	35
Chapter 5.	
Becoming your own Parent.	51
Chapter 6.	
Stress.	60
Chapter 7.	
Case Histories.	75
Chapter 8.	
Conclusions.	136
Appendix.	141
Glossary.	156
Bibliography.	160

The Author

Geoff Graham B.D.S. started using hypnosis in dentistry in 1960. He formed the Northern Counties Branch of The British Society of Medical and Dental Hypnosis in 1969. Since this time he has been involved in lecturing and running courses and workshops both in this country and Europe, North and South America, Australia, and the Far East. In 1972 he was made a Foreign Fellow of the American Society of Clinical Hypnosis. In 1973 while attending The Pan American Congress of Hypnosis in Brazil he was made a Member of Honour at that Conference. In 1974 he was made an Honorary Fellow of the Singapore Society of Clinical Hypnosis. He is a Founder Fellow of the British Society of Medical and Dental Hypnosis and has acted as a National Assessor for the Certificate of Accreditation issued by that society and possesses a Certificate in his own right.

He has spent over a year attending part-time training as a Primal Therapist with the International Society of Primal Therapists organized by Dr. W. Swartley. Although he is not a hospital consultant both B.U.P.A. and P.P.P. accept Geoff Graham on a consultant basis when patients are referred to him by other Hospital Consultants. He has now treated well over two thousand patients with hypnosis, most of whom have been referred to him. He is also a member of the International Society of Hypnosis.

He feels many patients seeking help with psychological problems get very little real help, and has written this book to make the information and experience he has had the privilege to obtain from patients, available both to therapists, but more importantly to the intelligent public so that they may be in a position to help themselves, with the carefully structured self-help exercises outlined in this book.

Acknowledgments

I would like to offer my sincere thanks to all those who have helped me produce this book, especially to Elizabeth who was responsible for the first and subsequent editings. Also thanks are due to Michael and Peter who read through the manuscript and gave most valuable advice, on both the content, and presentation. Mostly, I would like to thank and dedicate this book to my patients, who have taught me more than anyone, both with the theory and the treatment outlined in this book. Without them there would be no book.

Introduction

CAN YOU CUDDLE YOUR PARENTS AFFECTIONATELY? Twenty-five years experience of treating a wide range of neurotic patients, particularly those suffering from extreme phobias or excessive feelings of anger or guilt, has taught me the importance of that interesting and fundamental question. I have yet to meet anyone suffering from the above conditions who can cuddle both parents. It may be that one parent was absent, or one or both parents were not that sort. No matter what the reason, the neurotic is unable to perform the simple task of taking their parents and holding them warmly.

It is my belief that, to grow up safely, every child needs a warm, safe, loving environment that is shown to all the family. If this is not the case then the child hurts, and even if the child is not aware of what it is missing, its behaviour will be affected. To receive love is to have contact in three ways, physically, emotionally and intellectually. If these three contacts are not made and felt by the child then, it is my firm belief, a part of the child's psyche is arrested in its development and remains child-like in the grown adult. This causes the adult to behave immaturely and when the unconscious mind recognizes the irrationality of this behaviour, the person will feel anxiety, anger or guilt.

Jinnie Jefferies, who works with some of the most violent prisoners at Grendon Psychiatric Prison in England, reporting to Sheila Duncan in *The Sunday Times*, 11 November 1984 stated that, the longer she works with these men, the more convinced she becomes that the bitterness and pain of severely deprived childhoods are always at the bottom of crimes of terrible violence. She goes on to say that when these fearsome figures are reduced to tears during treatment, they all show a hunger for warmth: the sort of comfort and cuddles they never received from their parents. Sometimes the tears are the recognition of the hurt bestowed on them by brutal fathers or rejecting mothers.

Everyone has their own way of handling the hurt of not feeling loved as a child. If they cannot cuddle their parents then a part of their mind has not grown-up. One of the best ways to help that part to grow and mature is to find a way of giving it the love and understanding it never had during childhood, so that it can grow up in a safe environment. Who better to do that than the patients themselves? Who knows better than the patients what they didn't have, when they were small, and what they would have liked to have had? If they can only find a way to help that part of their mind to mature and become as old as they are chronologically, then they have more options in their behaviour and life. The purpose of this book is to outline ways of doing that, using various exercises aimed at developing the mind's capacity to overcome previous conditioning. The point of treatment is to give you more options in life. Who better to become the parent you never had than you yourself?

In this book case histories have been quoted to demonstrate the problems presented by patients. The names and personal details of those patients have been changed slightly to protect individual identities. The treatments used in these cases illustrate the application of my theories and ideas. These theories and ideas have been developed while treating thousands of patients over twenty-five years. They are partly what fits, partly what patients offer as explanations for their behaviour. They are not claimed to be proven facts. You may not feel they offer any new insight into the extremes of Fear, Anger and Guilt. However you may come to believe, as I do, that we can help ourselves and out patients by using the theories described in this book. By selling these ideas to my own patients, I find they become conscious of having many more options in their lives. The journey of life itself becomes more enjoyable and that's what life is all about.

Geoff Graham.
July 1985.

CHAPTER 1

"The Marathon and The Purpose of Life Itself"

Hypnosis can be thought of as a state of mind where there is a marked narrowing in the field of concentration with a corresponding increase in attention within that field. Consequently if you enter a state of hypnosis, whatever is said to you while you are in that altered state is more likely to get maximum attention. It is therefore very useful when doing the exercises described in this book to first enter this altered state we call hypnosis. When you are in hypnosis you do not feel very different at all, and you may not realize you are hypnotized. That is of little importance; what is important is that whatever is said to you, either by a hypnotist, or by yourself, to yourself as in auto-hypnosis, is accepted and acted upon more strongly than it would be if you were not in this altered state. It is not essential to go into hypnosis to do the exercises which follow, but you will find they work more quickly and more effectively while under hypnosis. Therefore the first exercise in this book is to find a way to enter hypnosis quickly and easily by yourself.

EXERCISE 1. Find a comfortable chair preferably with a high back which will support your head. Sit comfortably in the chair and rest your head on the back. Place your feet with your soles flat on the ground. At this point I always suggest that female patients remove their shoes. Ladies tend to take off their shoes when returning home after work, a shopping expedition, an evening out etc. and it is therefore a major aid to their relaxation. Place both your arms comfortably and lightly on each armrest of the chair; if there are no armrests on the chair, place one hand upon each knee. Do not fold your arms or clasp your hands, as both these behaviours are defensive. Look straight ahead of you then, without altering the position of your head, turn your eyes up to look towards your eyebrows. Turn them up as high as you can without moving your head. Keeping your eyes turned up close your eyes. (SPIEGEL'S EYEROLL INDUCTION) (1).

Now relax your eyes, let them become so relaxed, so heavy they feel they just won't open, and hang on to that feeling. Now let that feeling spread through the whole of your body. Let your body sink comfortably down into the chair. (ELMAN DEEPENING) (2).

While your body is sinking down into the chair turn your mind inward to look at your mind. (GEOFF GRAHAM & N. L. P.) Let your mind feel as if it can float. (SPIEGEL) (3).

While your body is sinking comfortably into the chair and your mind is pleasantly floating, turn your thoughts to something that gives you great pleasure and joy. Let yourself enjoy that feeling as much as you can. Hang on to that good feeling and imagine how good it would be to be wide awake with your eyes wide open with that good feeling. (GEOFF GRAHAM'S SCRAP BOOK) (4). Now open your eyes and be wide awake with that good feeling.

End of first exercise. Repeat this exercise until it becomes easy and quick to feel relaxed and comfortable with a good feeling about something of your own choice.

The Marathon

Now that you have practised entering a heightened state of concentration I would like to tell you a true story about yourself. Perhaps the most common induction to this heightened state is four words. Those words are ONCE UPON A TIME. If you say 'once upon a time' to a child, giants, fairies, and beanstalks going right up into the sky all become a possibility. If you say 'once upon a time' to an adult, late at night, with the wind howling outside, a late horror film on the T.V., many adults may look in the cupboard or under the bed, just in case. So if 'once upon a time' is an induction technique I say to you all, "ONCE UPON A TIME . . . each and every one of you were released with fifty million others in the birth canal and you ran a marathon race. The size you were and the distance you had to travel is equivalent to you now running a marathon race against fifty million. You ran, you swam, you pushed, you shoved and you fought against fifty million others, with no one to help you, and you won. You proved that you were the fittest to survive. You reached the ovum and succeeded in penetrating it and uniting the genes you had carried up the birth canal with the genes of the ovum. You created your life, therefore YOU ASKED TO BE HERE." (See the second exercise, below.)

Some ladies have difficulty in associating themselves with a sperm. I say to them "it is the sperm which carries the sex gene to the ovum. Their sperm was all female, and won that marathon, and created their lives, making it the race of their life: they are the only one to survive in that race".

I would also like to point that there isn't anyone else here on this earth for any other reason than that, SO YOU HAVE JUST AS MUCH RIGHT AS ANY OTHER PERSON TO BE HERE. (See the third exercise, below.) When we created our own lives by entering the ovum and uniting the genes, we started on the journey of life.

The Journey of Life

The first part of that journey was in growing. That single cell divided into two, then four, then eight, sixteen, thirty two, sixty four, one hundred and twenty eight and so on, until they were made up of millions of cells; that single cell gave to each cell the same genes that made them what they are. Those genes knew how they should look, the colour of their eyes and hair and skin, the shape of their face, mouth, teeth, size of hands, feet and everything about them. Those genes could also remember how they succeeded in winning that marathon race to be here. YOU CAN WIN AND BE A SUCCESS. (See the fourth exercise, below.) It is my belief that it is this cellular memory of success and the bliss feeling after conception which unconsciously promotes people to enter marathon races today. If a marathon race is announced in my part of the world, thousands of people put down their names to participate. We all know it is a painful thing to run a marathon, and yet thousands of people rush to take part. If you ask, most of them haven't got any idea why they are going to try to do it. Many of them will admit to getting a 'high feeling' from doing it. The same as conception. It is that cellular memory that promotes them to enter quite unconsciously. If that memory is there then we ought to be able to find it without having to run a marathon.

Various things happen to us during the journey of life which teach us behaviour and modify the way we feel. Most of the unpleasant things we learn seem to reduce our options in life. The remainder of this book consists of a review of those unpleasant things which limit our options, and how we may overcome those limits and increase our options. Unfortunately no book could cover all of the learning patterns of life, so this one must only be an overview.

The Ultimate Destination

From the moment of conception there is only one thing certain on the journey through life, and that is someday we will reach the end of our journey and die. I would like you to contemplate the possibilities of that end and what may be next. I would like to discuss with you three possibilities at the end of your journey. The first possibility is that when you die you are either burnt, or buried, and that's the end of it; but if that is all life is about then it makes a nonsense of the very structure and organization of life itself, so I would like you to contemplate another possibility.

The second possibility is that when you die you move on to whatever is next; but if we all move on to whatever is next then why do some people have such a hard time trying to make the first journey? Why can't we all just go straight to whatever is next? So I would like to give you a third possibility, and I stress that this third possibility is the only one worth contemplating even if it is wrong.

The third possibility is that this journey is a journey to raise our consciousness to a higher plane. To mature, and find a way of overcoming our difficulties, to become responsible for

THE MARATHON AND THE PURPOSE OF LIFE ITSELF 7

ourselves and stop playing the 'Blame Game'. Every feeling we have is a personal experience which we manufacture for ourselves and we alone are responsible for how we feel. However if we start blaming other people or other things for how we feel, then we are playing the 'Blame Game'. Most of us play the 'blame game'; we are taught to play it when we are very young. Once we have started blaming others for the way we feel, the only way out of those feelings is to change the people or things we think are to blame. But that option is often impossible so we become trapped within those feelings. I saw a very good example of the 'blame game' being played when I visited some friends. They have a young daughter of just one year old. One day while she was learning to walk and was still a little unsteady on her feet, she staggered across the room, bumped into a table and fell to the ground crying. Much to my amazement both her parents rushed to her and started to smack the table saying "naughty table". This distracted the child and she stopped crying and began to laugh. I said *"Hang on a minute what about the table? perhaps it is hurting, and after all it didn't move so it could hardly be its fault"*. They didn't see what I was getting at, protesting that their ploy had worked; the child had stopped crying and had even begun to laugh. I left it at that until about twenty minutes later the little girl again staggered across the room, this time bumping into her father's leg. Once again she fell to the ground crying. I called *"naughty father"*, who only then realised what I had been talking about earlier. Seeing that their earlier behaviour had made him the bad guy, he bent down and picked his daughter up, to clean up the mess his earlier behaviour had made. His daughter, however, had learned well and this was naughty Daddy who was now picking her up, so she cried even louder and looked pleadingly at Mother saying with her eyes "come and take me off this beast". Her mother, reading the child absolutely correctly, rushed across the room and pulled the girl from her dad. So I now explained that mother's behaviour had just wiped dad out, and confirmed he was the bad guy. He, realizing that what I had just said was correct, grabbed the child back saying "let me clean up my mess", and the baby cried even louder. Mother grabbed her back again and she by this time being thoroughly confused, cried even louder. Mother and father argued that night and again in the morning. Playing the "blame game" had confused the child and created a void between mother and father which neither of them had the necessary skill to cross.

The purpose of life is to mature and stop playing the "blame game" and become responsible for self, thus raising one's consciousness to a higher plane. The difficulties we encounter on the journey are tests to see if we are succeeding. If we succeed in raising our consciousness to that higher plane then we move on to that higher level after death, but if we don't then we are just recycled to do it all over again. This is the only possibility worth contemplating, even if it's wrong; because if we accept it then we have a purpose in life: to overcome our difficulties and make it to that higher plane so when we die we can move on to that better level. If, when we die, there is no better level we won't be around to be disappointed, but at least we will have made the most of this life. Surely that is the purpose of life itself, to make the most of it. (See fifth exercise; I WILL OVERCOME MY DIFFICULTIES AND I WILL BECOME RESPONSIBLE FOR MYSELF, below.)

It is most important we should accept the statement that if we don't achieve that higher plane we are just recycled to do it all over again, because this gives us that most important motive to try even harder to make it. I had a patient who was contemplating suicide and said to me at the next visit after I had told her about the recycling, "Damn you, Graham, I can't even get out of it that way now can I?" I just shook my head and said *"No"*. So you see why this third option is the only one worth considering, even if it's wrong.

Security

The first nine months on the journey of life form a period when most of us are loved, needed, necessary and wanted, and have everything supplied to us without asking for it. This is what real love is; to have one's real needs supplied without having to ask for anything. Loving someone is to be aware of

THE MARATHON AND THE PURPOSE OF LIFE ITSELF

their real needs (not neurotic needs) and satisfying them, if necessary to the detriment of your own. Throughout the first nine months of your life you are, in all probability, growing blissfully in the womb. During that stage of your development you have a dual consciousness, that of yourself, and a common consciousness with your mother because at that time you are also part of your mother.

When I touch myself I am O.K., I feel safe, secure, and in close contact everywhere. When I touch the womb I feel O.K. and that is part of me too. (COMMOM CONSCIOUSNESS.) So touching me I'm O.K. Touching the womb, I'm also O.K. But the womb is everywhere so I'm O.K. everywhere. The womb is my world but I am the world. (COSMIC CONSCIOUSNESS.) It's like, 'I am a pebble on the beach but I am also the beach'. This feeling of being O.K. and the world's O.K. is a gut feeling that is security.

When you get out of the womb, you realise that your world has increased and now includes other people. Security then becomes a gut feeling of 'I'm O.K., you're O.K. and the world's O.K. Security is a feeling which is remembered from the womb but it has to be reinforced outside the womb. You need to feel loved, to be held and cuddled by both parents, to be given all the contact you need and to have your real needs satisfied. Without these things, you sense constant insecurity outside the womb. You search in vain for security and you never feel any better. If you don't feel secure, parts of your mind cannot grow up and mature. You will never reach a higher plane of consciousness unless you find a way of feeling secure. The only way you can do that is by becoming the parent you never had.

There are circumstances in which you may spend the first nine months of your life, in the womb, feeling that you are unwanted and unloved. You grow up outside the womb with feelings of unworthiness, wishing you weren't here. For you too, the only way to overcome those feelings is to become the parent you never had and to give yourself the feeling of being wanted and loved. The following exercises are intended to help you become your own parent.

EXERCISE 2.   Before doing all these exercises it is better to enter that heightened state of concentration described in exercise 1, up to the part where you turn your mind inwards to look at your mind. While you are looking at your mind, contemplate that marathon you ran to be here and tell yourself that by winning that race YOU ASKED TO BE HERE.

EXERCISE 3.   While you are in that heightened state of consciousness and thinking about having asked to be here, remember that there is no-one on this earth for any other reason than winning a marathon. Therefore tell yourself, YOU HAVE JUST AS MUCH RIGHT AS ANY OTHER PERSON TO BE HERE.

EXERCISE 4.   By winning that marathon race you proved that you were the fittest of fifty million to survive, and you have the right to take the journey through life and win. So tell yourself, YOU CAN WIN AND BE A SUCCESS AND RAISE YOUR CONSCIOUSNESS TO THAT HIGHER PLANE.

EXERCISE 5.   Tell yourself YOU WILL WIN SO THAT YOU WON'T HAVE TO DO IT ALL OVER AGAIN, AND WILL BECOME RESPONSIBLE FOR YOURSELF.

EXERCISE 6.   YOU LIKE YOURSELF FOR WINNING A MARATHON AND YOU WILL LEARN TO LOVE YOURSELF.

You should spend no more than two to three minutes at a time doing the exercises in this book because you cannot hold the level of concentration necessary to do them correctly for more time than that. Repeat the exercises every two to three hours until you begin to feel what you are telling yourself, and repeat again if you lose that feeling.

CHAPTER 2

Behaviour at Birth—Negative Imprinting —First Line Trauma

There are three known psychological methods of learning in life, according to R. R. TILLEARD-COLE.

The first of these is IMPRINTING. Imprinting occurs at conception, in inter-uterine life and especially at birth and during the first few hours after birth, and at any subsequent time when the stimulus is sufficiently extreme to make it a 'once and for all' learning experience. An example of this method of learning is that if a child puts its hand in a fire and burns itself it will tend to recoil from heat for a long time afterwards.

The second method of learning is PAVLOVIAN CONDITIONING. This method requires a large amount of reinforcement by repeating the stimulus frequently over a short period of time. Pavlov demonstrated this method by feeding dogs and at the same time ringing a bell. After something like two to three weeks he found that he could ring the bell without feeding the dogs, and they would salivate excessively, as if they were being fed. This effect would wear off fairly quickly if not again reinforced. In life, if the stimulus is repeatedly reinforced, like a parent not being able to show a child love and affection, it is most probable that the child will grow up having most of its emotional behaviour blunted, perverted or deviant.

The third method of learning is OPERANT CONDITIONING. This method is nearly always goal-related. If there is a reward after doing something, and that reward is positive, we soon learn to do it again in the hope of getting another reward. It is, however, equally important when the reward is negative; when a child gets smacked for doing something, it soon learns either not to do it, or not get found out. This having to 'not get found out' is the source of our first lies. To survive, we must try to get love from our parents. To do this, we often have to forget who, and what we are. What we want for ourselves often is totally opposite to that which our parents want for us, and so we lose our identity and self-confidence, no longer trusting our thoughts or feelings. We begin to do one thing and feel another. This inner conflict is the birth and cause of all neurosis, fear, anger and guilt.

Neurotics do not think and feel the same thing at the same time. Their feelings are not 'REAL' or relevant to the present, with true concepts of the here and now. They have a faulty perception on the 'feeling' side of the brain and of the here and now. For examples see the following table:

COMPLAINT	THINK	FEEL
Agoraphobia*	I am not any safer in the house and I should be able to go into the supermarket.	Frightened when I go to the door and terrified in the supermarket. I 'must get out' and go home.
Compulsive handwasher	I know it is silly.	I must keep washing them or I feel very uncomfortable.
Alcoholic	I know I should not drink.	I must have another drink, I can't stop.
Smoking	I know it is harmful and causes cancer and will kill me.	I must have another cigarette.
Reactive depression	I know worrying about it isn't going to help.	I can't get it out of my mind.

*Note: Most people who suffer from agoraphobia also suffer from claustrophobia, and vice versa, because the former naturally follows the latter at birth. First of all they are claustrophobic in the birth canal, and then they are so terrified by the time they get out that even being 'OUT' is terrifying. Agoraphobia is born out of the left-over feelings from the claustrophobia. It is the anticipation of what happened on the way out that makes 'out' frightening.

At conception, inter-uterine life, and especially birth and for the first few hours after birth, most of the learning experiences are sufficiently extreme as to be a one-off experience or IMPRINT learning of behaviour.

What is the evidence that birth has any effect on our behaviour? Freud claimed that birth was our first trauma and the origin of all the anxieties at the root of later psychological problems. He said that later traumas were all, in some sense, a repetition and reinforcement of that first birth experience. He claimed that we learnt to block off from consciousness the primary anxiety at birth, thus causing a cutting off or disconnecting of oneself from the feelings of anxiety at birth, leaving in one a disconnected fear that later manifests itself as free-floating anxiety. Thus the displaced emotion from birth sets the pattern for all later reactions to anxiety, building up more free-floating anxiety which then reduces our options in life.

Rank in his book The Trauma of Birth built upon Freud's work and hypothesized that all neurosis originated at birth. Ferenczi extended and deepened Rankian birth theory. Frederic Leboyer, David Cheek, Frank Lake, Lewis Mehl and many others all add further evidence of the effect of birth on subsequent behaviour.

Stanislav Grof, in working with deep regression assisted by the drug LSD, formulated the FOUR PERINATAL MATRICES OF CONSCIOUSNESS developed from inter-uterine life and birth.

The first one he called 'Symbiotic Unity'. This develops from inter-uterine experiences leading to feelings of security, protection, satisfaction and cosmic unity (see previous chapter on security). This gives rise to our first basic primal anchor feeling. (See the seventh exercise in this book, SECURITY IS A GUT FEELING OF BEING LOVED).

The second matrix he called 'Antagonism'. This resulted from the reactions to the onset of the contractions of birth. These give rise to feelings of claustrophobia, physical torment, existential crisis and helplessness, mixed with feelings of guilt. These experiences, I believe, lead in later life to the behaviour of claustrophobia, 'I have got to get out of here', in church, buses, theatres, crowded pubs, supermarkets: it is the cash-out desks they have got to go through in supermarkets that triggers 'I have got to get out'. At the dentists, lying flat in the dentist's chair, surrounded by equipment and people who are going to hurt me, unable to help myself in any way gives rise to the feeling 'I must get out of here' or avoid this situation. Such a person is the classic dental phobic. These feelings of 'I must get out of here' will arise in any crowded place where I may get hurt or be unable to help myself or get out easily, like a plane etc. The feelings of guilt built up from 'I should not be here', or even 'I should not be alive', which gives rise of the behaviour of suicide, or fear of death or of illness leading to death.

The third stage Grof called 'Synergism'. This stage starts at the beginning of propulsion through the birth canal. The struggle for survival counters the threat of suffocation or being crushed. The effect it has on behaviour, like at any stage during the birth, depends on the severity of the experience at that point in time. Each moment of the birth is a unique experience, possibly leading to a different behaviour. I am sure in my own mind that depression is a learnt behaviour from this stage of the birth when one's head is through the pelvic arch and one's shoulders are stuck. We are at the point of no return where, if we cannot go forwards or backwards, the only behaviour we have left to us is to stop feeling. At the same time we are threatened by negative feelings and, if no progress is made, become frightened to feel again. This to my mind, is the birth of classical depression. This stage may also give rise to the 'wipe out' feelings of 'they are trying to get rid of me', which lead to the baby rejecting its mother. ("After all she tried to get rid, or worse kill, me so why should I ever trust her again. If I can't trust my mother how can I ever trust anyone again?") This, leads to the classical case of a person who cannot trust anyone and has no choice in the matter. If the baby rejects its mother because of a 'wipe out', mother may learn not to cuddle the child, not because she doesn't want to, or because she can't, but because the child has rejected her and refuses to be cuddled. Nevertheless the child will eventually live to regret the day it rejected her, as the effect will be the same as if the mother couldn't love the child.

A patient who was a persistent bed-wetter was brought to me by his mother. She told me that her son had a very difficult birth and every time she tried to pick him up the infant was violently sick and screamed his head off. She was told eventually that the baby must be allergic to her and not to pick him up. He was taken away to be fed and his mother stopped making any physical contact with him. This eventually ended up in neither of them being able to show each other any physical love.

The fourth stage of Grof's matrices is called 'Separation'. This is a feeling of relief and relaxation and independence, mixed, however, with a fear of being alone and often exhaustion. If, however, the baby has stopped feeling in the previous stage and doesn't feel it has got 'out' this will lead to a demanding feeling of dependence and will greatly reduce one's options in life. This leads to the 'psychological vampire' patient who goes round plugging in to people, draining them of any succour and then moving on the the next, to do the same all over again.

Janov and his primal therapy says that feelings that are too painful to intergrate and accept, are suppressed and remain in the system as reverberating circuits, threatening to be felt for ever. These unfelt feelings keep attaching themselves by projecting on to the present making our current feelings unreal and fearful and painful.

Janov also says that the only treatment for that pain is to feel it. This may, however, just reinforce the original trauma and make it worse. It is also playing the 'blame game' which as we have already seen, can be a very dangerous game to play. I feel that one of the main dangers in primal therapy is that the patient may get stuck in a negative primal and try to go on feeling it until it's all felt, long after it has been felt. (They just feel they cannot get out of the feeling, another birth behaviour).

The imprinted behaviour learned at birth and for the first few hours afterwards correspond to Janov's First Line Traumas. They are often life and death situations. Let us look at some of the behaviours learned at birth, and the organs they affect. Naturally they affect the organs which are fully innovated and working at the time of birth.

Migraine

In my opinion migraine is always a learned birth behaviour. Let us look at what happens at birth to our intra-cranial pressure. In order to allow our head to pass through the birth canal we reduce our intra-cranial pressure. This allows the cranial plates of bone which are not united at birth, to come closer together, and if necessary to overlap, thus making our head smaller, and easier to pass through the pelvic arch and birth canal. Having got our head out we then reflate the pressure to restore the shape. This may be a life saving procedure, which some of our minds remember. Migraine sufferers do just that at times of stress. While the stress is active as a result of learned behaviour they reduce their intra-cranial pressure giving rise to the visual signs (flashing lights etc) and nausea, then when the stress is over for example at the weekends or on awakening, there is increased intra-cranial pressure giving rise to the blinding headache. Unfortunately for migraine sufferers, the skull plates are fully united long before the symptoms occur, and the method used by our minds to overcome the problem of stress has itself become the problem. The logical treatment of migraine therefore is to reframe the behaviour regarding the intra-cranial pressure. We do this by having the patient enter the state of heightened concentration and turning the mind inwards to find that part of the mind which at birth saved their life by changing the pressure in the head, and thanking it for doing so, but then carefully reminding it that what saved their life at birth has now become the problem. As the circumstances are now different, to first decrease and then increase the pressure in the head does not help the sufferer to cope with the stress but may make it worse. It is a negative behaviour which may force the patient to opt out and although he may feel better after the attack, there are much better ways of handling stress. Ask that part of the mind which is responsible for the migraine to find a better way of helping to cope with stress than giving you a headache. It is also often necessary to work on the negative anchors involved in the migraine.

Negative anchors are those times and situations in which you generally have a negative behaviour. For instance a professional colleague of mine came to ask me to help him stop smoking. After the session was over we decided to go over the road to have a drink in the local pub, and discuss old times. On entering the pub my friend said to me "this damn pub is making me want a cigarette; I don't really want one but I usually have one when I go for a drink". The pub was the negative anchor. It is often necessary, but fortunately fairly easy, to neutralize the negative anchors surrounding a behaviour. Each time the patient resists the anchor it becomes weaker. I was treating a migraine patient who woke up every morning with a headache, consequently she used to dread going to bed because she knew she would wake with the headache. She was programming herself every night to have that headache. It was essential in her case to reframe that dread so she could go to bed expecting to have a restful night's sleep and to awake feeling refreshed and very clear-headed. I got her mind to change that dread to a pleasant expectation, by the process of reframing (See chapter 6 on reframing).

Other birth imprinted behaviour may result from the excessive fear the baby experiences during the birth. This may take the form of panic attacks in crowded places etc., in palpitations or missed heart beats or imagined heart attacks. Claustrophobia and agoraphobia are both learned birth behaviours. After all the first opens space we meet is the world we encounter when we leave the womb. (See Operant Conditioning at the beginning of this chapter.) A patient came to me to be helped with her agoraphobia. She told me that whenever she went to go out of the door of her home, she feared she would be drowned in water. She said she couldn't understand this, as there was no water, for miles, round her house. There was, however, lot of amniotic fluid in the birth canal in which she nearly drowned.

The baby being born may try to suppress the excessive fear it is experiencing during the birth, in tension. This tension may be held in the organs which are in full use at the time of birth, like the heart or the lungs, giving rise to the behaviour of asthma or some speech difficulties, or the stomach producing the behaviour of holding tension into the stomach lining causing ulcers. Tension may be held in the colon leading to spastic colon.

Some special difficulties may occur during the birth, for instance, with the cord. During the best part of nine months the cord is your friend and provider, and first sex object. A scan of the developing baby may often show the baby playing with the cord. During the birth, however, the cord may become your enemy, getting in the way or cutting the oxygen off, getting round your neck and threatening to strangle you. This may lead to certain speech difficulties, to respiratory difficulties, to choking feelings or to swallowing difficulties. Anorexia Nervosa may have its roots in cord trouble at birth. What was your friend and provider for nine months may suddenly become your worst enemy, giving rise to love-hate feelings in later life. Anorexic patients may have such trouble with the cord during the birth that afterwards when the cord is cut and the throat and stomach become the provider, they have to reject them. Somehow this is also mixed up with mother as well. They become dependent on mother and at the same time reject her and so set out to punish her by not eating. Guilt plays a big part in this feeling. There is often an unconscious feeling of 'I should not be here' and if I eat I will grow up and have to be here, but if I don't eat I won't grow and won't have to become responsible. The treatment is to teach them that they asked to be here and they may as well make the most of the journey otherwise they will just have to do it all over again. At the same time it is necessary to help them to have a more accurate body image of themselves. Reframing of various parts of the mind involved in negative behaviour in the anorexic is also necessary.

The feeling of loneliness is also often associated with cord loss. Little boys find a little piece of cord remains a little lower down in the form of the penis and they play with that. Lonely people often feel incomplete and need something to be a cord substitution. The only truly happy people are those who have become their own provider and take full responsibility for themselves and have fully reached adult maturity. This surely, is the very purpose of life itself.

A simple test for cord trauma, is to take a piece of inch rubber tubing about two feet long, and place it round the patient's neck and vibrate it quickly. Most patients who have had a cord problem at birth will find this quite intolerable. Most of them will not like anything tight round their neck, like a polo-necked sweater etc.

Particular Difficulties at Birth

There are a number of special difficulties associated with birth that lead to particular behaviour imprinting.

1. Forceps Delivery.

Babies who are helped out with forceps tend to seek out dependency situations in later life and then resent that dependency. They suffer many more headache situations and have a higher degree of mental illness, neurosis and have a much greater tendency to intellectualise. External controls or attitudes become over-important in the day to day life situations. They also have a much greater feeling of "wipe out" and therefore suffer from more guilt of being here.

2. Delayed Births.

Babies who suffer delayed births or long births tend to resent delays in later life. They get impatient, unreasonable and uncomfortable if kept waiting and will often walk away from such situations.

3. Multiple Births.

These involve many more complications in later life. The conflict often starts in the womb for space and for getting out first. A patient of mine, who was a twin, could not look at a particular picture of a pair of twins in the womb. It made him feel violently sick. (Suppression of the pain he felt in that conflict, into the stomach lining, making him feel sick. If he can feel sick just looking at a picture, then the dynamic processes of that conflict of there being two of them in the womb at the same time, is still affecting him now.) He is also likely to choose his stomach lining to repress tension in the future. (Learned behaviour.)

4.   Breech Birth.

The major risk in breech births is that as the body comes through the cervix, the head gets caught and the baby can suffer from oxygen starvation due to cord blocking. I had a patient, called Tom, who was sent to me from a psychiatrist friend with a possible diagnosis of schizophrenia. Tom experienced many unreal feelings one of which was a feeling he got in shops or similar places where people were serving him behind a counter. If their hands went under the counter he was convinced they were going to get something that would knock his head off, so if this happened he would have to run away. He also felt as if he lived in his head and had no connection with his body. During therapy, I discovered he was a breech birth. When we, (treatment is always a contract between patient and therapist and both are involved in the experience), had him review his birth in an altered state he abreacted and screamed, "they are pulling my head off. The buggers are trying to kill me!" As you can imagine he was quite unable to trust anyone. How can you trust anyone if your own mother tried to kill you by getting someone to pull your head off at birth. In therapy I had him disassociate his mind from his body and watch his own birth as if it were a film. I asked him to take his mind to the baby and convince the baby that the breech birth was an unfortunate mistake on his part and everyone concerned with the birth was trying to get him out safely. Everyone concerned wanted him safe, healthy and alive, and no one wanted to kill him. They also succeeded in getting him out alive and healthy so he need never again fear 'they will try to have my head off'. (See also the section in chapter 5 on becoming your own parent). I also had him review that screen many times by himself and he eventually began to believe it and lost his fear of people behind counters. I also had to do some work to make him reconnect the feelings between his head and his body and he now has many more options in life. I hope you can now see how difficult births can greatly reduce our options.

Perhaps you might think, "So why don't we all have Caesarean births?" Unfortunately they have their difficulties too. Babies born by Caesarean section do not feel the contractions of the womb and do not learn to struggle to get out, so they have a great tendency to quit when things get tough later in life. They do not know how to fight to attain goals as they never learned to do that at birth. Often they are furious at being plucked out of the comfort of the womb and have difficulty in identifying 'Self'. They tend to be short tempered and quit when the going gets tough. They blame the world and everyone else for any failures. Responsibility is something they have great difficulty with, so they are most frustrated in their journey through life. Therapy entails the patient going through an enacted normal birth and learning to struggle to get out.

Not all births are traumatic but many are. When they are, because of a total lack of previous experience, the child suffers extremes of anxiety and fear. Even as adults one of the most common fears is of the unknown. When birth traumas do occur they are probably intensified, much more unexpected and therefore much more distorted and misunderstood, hence the gross distortion in the behaviour imprinting. If a baby chooses a response learned at birth because of the imprinting, that behaviour becomes reinforced so that by the time it is an adult many of its responses are either birth responses or modified birth responses.

Post Natal Depression

A mother giving birth to a child will frequently unconsciously relive parts of her own birth with many of her own birth feelings. If she had to stop feeling during her own birth the reliving of that may reinforce that imprinted behaviour and trigger off the depression. Hence her inability to enjoy the birth of her new baby. She will be unable to bond with the child and may find, much to her annoyance, she cannot accept the child. This can be most distressing both for the mother and the child.

Bonding

Immediately following the birth it is essential that the child is bonded with at least one of its parents. This occurs when eye to eye contact is made between the parent and the child while the parent is thinking and feeling how wonderful the child is. If this does not occur, the child will grow up unable to make that eye to eye contact with anyone without feeling uncomfortable. I have a friend who almost immediately after he was born was placed in his cot, his father was so horrified by how he looked, because of his difficult birth, that the father recoiled and uttered, "My God!". He must have given my friend a terrible feeling because it has plagued him until fairly recently. The treatment for non-bonded people is to rebirth and establish a bond. (See exercise 24 chapter 5).

Many of the birth traumas are so excessive that it is necessary to work with a therapist first, before taking over control for yourself. Too much early pain results in almost total blocking out of reality, leaving the child, and later adult, insensitive to what is going on around them. This often leads to living in the head and not in touch with their real needs and feelings. (See examples in chapter 7.) The following exercises are not intended to replace an expert therapist but to assist and augment the therapy, where appropriate, between sessions.

Womb Return

Many people practice womb return, in bed or in the bath. It is not always a negative behaviour as it helps in clearing one's mind and collecting thoughts so that problem solving becomes much easier.

EXERCISE 7. While you are in that heightened state of concentration think about one or two of the good things about yourself, and celebrate those things by feeling good about them. It is essential you learn to celebrate things about yourself. At first you may have some difficulty in thinking good things about yourself because of a birth wipe out, but you must persevere until you can. Remember you must learn to love yourself so that others can, then you can feel secure because security is being loved.

EXERCISE 8.   Migraine sufferers. While in an altered state, find and thank the part of the mind that enabled you to make your head smaller at birth by first decreasing your intracranial pressure at a time of stress, and then reflating that pressure afterwards, but respectfully remind it that when your skull is firmly united this altering of pressure is no mature way of responding to stress. There are much better ways of responding to, and handling stress. (For these ways see chapter 6.) Ask it to try one or two of the more mature ways and give it the option. If that way doesn't work try another until one does, and you have no need then to have migraine.

EXERCISE 9.   Agoraphobics in an altered state must realise that the places in which they feel afraid are very different from the birth canal. After all, they did get out safely in the end. They do this by creating images of those places where they would normally want to get out of, and telling themselves that they will be able to get out quite easily when they need to, and until that time, they will enjoy where they are, and feel very safe there. You can create an image in many ways. You may be able to see it. If you can't, however, don't worry just think about it, and you will have a conceptual image. It is impossible to think about anything without forming some sort of image. Create that image in whichever way you normally think about things.

EXERCISE 10.   Asthmatics in an altered state create images of their breathing tubes relaxing and allowing the air to flow in, and particularly out, freely and easily. They see themselves taking control of their breathing and it becomes easier in all circumstances. Also learn some of the stress reducing exercises in chapter 6.

EXERCISE 11.   This exercise is for people suffering from guilt and a feeling of being a nuisance, or feeling they should not be here. People whose apologetic nature makes me call them 'Sorry-merchants'. In an altered state they must tell themselves that the purpose of life is to mature, otherwise they will just have to do it all over again. Have them create an image of being born, watching themselves experiencing that feeling of wipe out but reassuring themselves that every one concerned with the birth wants them to be alive, well, and get out easily. Have them reassure themselves that they did get out and it's over now and they need never feel like that again. They, and everyone else wanted them to be here, so there is no need to apologise.

EXERCISE 12.   If people haven't made a bond with a parent immediately following the birth, and have difficulty in looking people straight in the eyes without feeling uncomfortable, have them watch their own birth, and have them make eye to eye contact with themselves, as they are now, and themselves being born, while the adult self is thinking I love you and will help you to feel good.

This is the first step to becoming your own parent. (see chapter 5).

CHAPTER 3

From a few hours after birth to six years of age,—Negative Imprinting and Conditioning—Second Line Trauma—Cry for Attention

Most births are probably traumatic. After all, for the best part of nine months we experience being loved, being needed, being necessary and being wanted, and having everything supplied to us without having to ask for it. Then nature seems to deal us a blow as we meet our first difficulty, the first time we have to stuggle for anything: that struggle to get out.

Having looked at birth traumas and how they may affect us, why don't we all suffer from the symptoms? If both our parents can give back to us that feeling of being loved when we are out of the womb, and make us feel just as secure in the big world as we did in the womb, then the effects of the birth are minimized. Unfortunately, most parents are incapable of doing that, so many people suffer the symptoms. They suffer from those particular symptoms that belong to the behaviour learned at birth that they reinforce in later circumstances.

Let us look at some of the ways our parents fail us after the birth, when we are in the big world, what effect that has, and what we can do about it. For a start, it used to be a common practice not many years ago, and particularly after a difficult birth, for the baby to be removed from the mother to the baby ward, to allow the mother to recover and have a good night's sleep. The baby often screamed its head off, and is it any wonder after a difficult birth, after all the baby is only pounds to mothers stones, fourteen times more vulnerable, fourteen times more sensitive, everything that has happened is unknown, and much more likely to be misunderstood. The poor little mite all on its own, is left with very little choice but to try and shut off from its terror and pain. In doing so, it is reinforcing the behaviour of depression, learned at birth. It is also reinforcing the wipe out feeling, and the feeling of 'I should not be here', leading to guilt at being here. It forgets it asked to be here by winning a marathon, and blames its mother for having it. Once again it plays the 'blame game' and learns a new behaviour. Consequently, at a future time when things may get tough it will again play the 'blame game' and say "I didn't ask to be here". This means 'somebody, or something else, has to change, not me'. As it is most unlikely that anything else is going to change, this leaves the person with no options in life other than feeling more guilty for being here. It also increases the likelihood of the baby having to reject its own needs, such as the need to be loved, so it either rejects its mother, or becomes forever dependent on her. It cannot mature because it cannot get away from its dependence on her, or whoever it may have chosen as a substitute for her.

We see a lot of this in unsuitable marriages, in wife-bashing where the wife keeps going back for more, over and over again. We can see it in the meek little man who often is overpowered and dominated by some large, selfish wife. Wendy was a patient whose husband was a playboy who went out every night on his own. His wife had stopped going out with him on the rare occasions he invited her because he would still flirt with other women, even if Wendy was there. This hurt her so much that she would rather stay at home, than go out and have to witness his "Peter Pan" behaviour. In order to attempt to control him, she experienced acute panic attacks of such a nature that she would end up in hospital with a suspected heart attack, only to be told after all the tests, that there was nothing wrong with her. They prescribed tranquilisers for her which didn't really help, so she ended up with me. Shortly after meeting both her and her husband, I took her husband aside and told him that I felt she was being ill to try to control his selfish behaviour. I asked him if he felt he could change that behaviour in any way because if he could not, the only way I could help his wife would be to knock him off the pedestal she had put him on. He said "knock me off. I don't want to be responsible for her being ill". I asked him if he understood, and explained what that would mean if I did it, but he said "go ahead". I knocked him off fairly effectively and Wendy could not stand him, and left him. She eventually got a divorce, and was never more physically well, and subsequently married a more suitable man. The first husband became an alcoholic. If only one partner in a marriage is treated it often upsets the relationship, with the result that they may part. I have, however, never lost a marriage where both partners have had help. Where children are involved I believe every effort should be made to treat both partners.

When babies cry in their cot, or pram, or wherever, they need something. They are hurting, and want help. It may be that they are just lonely, but whatever that need, if it is not satisfied they hurt. If it is not satisfied by crying they will have to find another defence against that hurt. Perhaps they will just cry themselves to sleep. This is a common learned defence in adults, who at times of stress will go to sleep. This often is not a very successful defence, either in childhood or when adult, and the baby often has to try something else to get attention. One of the best ways to get attention, is to become ill. The child gets a tummy ache, or is sick, or wets, or fill its nappy. This often gets a response and once again a behaviour is learned. To get attention, be ill. Have a nappy rash, then mother will have to give me some attention. Older babies and children pull their hair out, and mother gets worried and pays attention.

A lady came to me, for help with a cancer phobia. I shall call her Pat. She had a friend once, and the two were inseperable, until the friend's mother got cancer. Her friend stopped seeing Pat because of her mother's illness and even after her friend's mother died, they never got together again. So her friend's mother got her daughter's attention by having cancer. Pat didn't feel loved as a child, so when she married she hoped to make up for all the love she had missed. Her husband's mother and sister didn't approve of her, and never came to see her. Her husband had some difficulty in showing her enough love, to make up for all the lack of love she had suffered. So Pat's mind thought of a way to get attention, probably a way she had found when she was very young and had consciously forgotten about. Her unconscious mind decided she had cancer; that would get her attention. Consciously she thought she had cancer and she told everybody, and they all paid attention, except the doctor, who along with the specialist, could find no trace of the disease. They told her there was nothing wrong with her, so she produced more symptoms. Pat had been told all about the symtoms of her particular cancer by another friend whose husband was a cancer specialist. However, the medical profession still could find no cancer in Pat, and told her so. She felt a little better, but when she began to realise what she had done to get attention she felt guilty. In one of the therapeutic sessions we had together, she said she was very naughty. At first she didn't know why, then all of this information came out. Now, because she had pretended to have cancer a year ago she believed she really had got it. This, however, was just her unconscious mind's way of relieving the guilt. The specialists and psychiatrists told her there was still nothing wrong with her, but she said they were not telling her the truth because they thought she could not take it. She had to believe that, or feel the guilt which was twice as bad now, because she had done it twice. 'Anyhow it would be worth it to see the look on my mother-in-law's and sister-in-law's faces when they are told I have cancer''. This last sentence, she also said while in a trance. That sentence however, also made her realise she was really just pretending again. We worked on the guilt, and how her mind was really just trying to get her the love she never had as a child, and it was really trying to help her in the only way it knew, at that time. I helped Pat's mind to see that it was a very poor way, and would never get her what she wanted. Her mind agreed, and we gave her some better options. The cure depends on how much she can handle and accept her guilt. At present she is still not convinced, because she hasn't learned to handle her guilt but I hope to work on that.

The unmet needs of young children manifest themselves either by the inability to show emotions and feelings in later life, or by being over emotionally demanding when adult, as in the example above. The patient has no option until she can mature.

Children must be allowed, and indeed encouraged, to show and express all their feelings, both positive and negative, when they are young. Otherwise they either become blunted for the rest of their lives, or develop into the classical Freudian hysteric, who is all emotion with nothing to focus it upon. I once had a patient who was in the depths of depression, was unable to show any feelings to anyone, or trust anyone. Her mother told me when she was very young she had very bad temper tantrums. She had been taken to a child psychiatrist who told her mother to lock her in her bedroom the next time she had a tantrum, and to repeat that every time until she stopped. She stopped having tantrums fairly quickly. Unfortunately she also stopped feeling for about twenty-nine years, until we reframed her defences.

If a child has to fend for itself because of lack of love during this early formative period, it often grows up defending against itself and its own needs. I had another patient, Bill, who was an alcoholic, who was married with two children. His wife was a very loving woman who loved her husband very much and wanted him to be loving in return. He wanted to be a family man, comfortable with his wife, son and daughter. However, he felt uncomfortable with his responsibility at home. It is what Bill wanted but he couldn't accept it. He had had to fend for himself, on his own, for the first twenty-odd years of his life, and responsibility now was just too much. When he went home he felt so uncomfortable he had first to get very drunk. He was very abusive to his wife and kept telling her that he was going to leave her. He was also abusive to his son, who unconsciously reminded him too much of himself, and his own very unhappy childhood. It was as though he had deliberately set out to destroy the one thing he had never had yet always wanted. It seemed that to accept the real love that was offered, was made too painful by the memory of the total lack of love in his childhood. To accept his real needs of "now" was made impossible, by feeling smothered by love from his wife and children, and he seemed to have no option but to reject them. This made him feel terribly guilty, so to live with himself he had to get even more drunk. He and his wife went to an alchoholic centre for treatment, and he was advised to leave home and live apart. This made Bill drink to drown his loneliness, so I told him to go back home and am helping him to cope with that, without feeling uncomfortable, by reframing his behaviour, so that it becomes closer to his needs. I am doing this by making him see what his real needs are, and asking his unconscious mind to change and try to help him to accept what he has always wanted. As he is much older now and the circumstances are such that he is much less likely to get hurt, it should be able to do that. In fact by refusing to accept his needs it is hurting both him and his family much more. The way his mind is trying to help him has become the problem so it needs to change.

At the early stages of our physical development the area being innovated is the skin and surface tissue, so any learned behaviour at that time seems to affect psychosomatically the skin and surface tissue. In later life, if the person chooses a second line learned behaviour as a defence to stress, or to get attention, then the area affected is the skin. Teenagers get spots, acne or eczema. Adults get psoriasis or alopecia. One of my patients who suffered from alopecia, took some persuading that she was doing it as a defence mechanism, but as soon as she accepted that, she began to get better and grow her hair back in again. Another patient who pulled her hair out by the handful stopped when she realised it was a regressive defence. Reframing the defence to a more mature behaviour was all that was required in both of these cases, along with Spiegel's split screen technique. (Exercise 13, below).

Joan was another patient who had psoriasis. After we worked with an ideo-motor finger control, (exercise 14, below) and found that her unconscious mind was trying to help her to get attention, she said to me in the waking state, "You know I do talk to everyone about my skin. I suppose I do get attention by it." We reframed her attention seeking and gave her more options to get what she wanted without having psoriasis. Joan's condition was so bad before treatment that every year she would have to go into hospital at least once, to have it treated with all sorts of ointments and creams. She has not been to hospital for two years now.

Children often start bedwetting, or get asthma, when another child is born into the family, as a means of getting the attention which they feel they have lost to their sibling. These are all negative defences which, if carried into adulthood, can be very restricting. A lady came to me for treatment for her asthma. Her husband enjoyed fell walking, but she wasn't so keen. She got very bad nocturnal asthma which prevented her going on the fell walks. When we reframed her excuses, her asthma cleared up. She also used Spiegel's split screen.

Adults produce tension headache as a "second line" defence against stress, by suppressing their mounting anxiety in the form of tension in the head, neck and shoulders, thus giving rise to the headache. The treatment of stress is discussed in chapter 6.

Being loved is to have all our needs satisfied without having to ask. We learn that in the womb; but many parents are incapable of giving love when we need it most, and so fail to establish a secure base from which we can go out into the world and mature. If we don't get that love and our emotions are blunted, the unsatisfied needs themselves will often decide for us what we will end up doing as a career. Unconsciously such people are pushed towards artistic outlets for their emotions. Many end up as actors acting out their emotions on stage, or artists painting their feelings, as a way of expressing themselves without having to take the blame for it. Their personal lives are often a disaster, and their children suffer the same fate, and follow their parents in their chosen profession for the same unconscious reasons.

EXERCISE 13.   SPIEGEL'S SPLIT SCREEN.
First of all, use auto-hypnosis to enter a special state of heightened concentration. When you begin to feel you mind comfortably floating as if it were free, imagine a cinema, or

television, screen, divided down the middle, on the wall in front of you. If you can see it, so much the better, but if you can't just think about it as a conceptual image. You don't have to see it for this technique to work. While you have the image of the screen on the other side of the room, see (either visually or conceptually) the behaviour you would like to change on one half of the screen. Now see the behaviour you would like to have to replace the unwanted one on the other side of the screen. Choose which behaviour you want and tell your mind. Having chosen, bring back from the screen the behaviour you would like, leaving the one you don't want on the other side of the room. Integrate the desired behaviour with your mind by thinking how good it would be to have that desired behaviour (see operant conditioning in the second chapter), and how you would feel doing it. (Teaching you to feel real feelings again). Integrate your mind with your body, open your eyes and go and adopt the desired behaviour.

With the three cases described in this chapter, the alopecia patient saw her hair falling out on one side of the screen and it growing back in again strong and healthy on the other. The hair pulling one saw herself pulling her hair out by the handful on one side, and leaving her hair to grow strong and healthy on the other. In both these cases, their hair grew back healthy and strong. With the asthmatic, she saw herself breathing with great difficulty on one side, and breathing easily and effortlessly on the other. Her asthma got better and better. As the improvement is made you see the two images becoming the same. What you do and what you would like to do become the same, then you only need one image.

This technique can be used to change any behaviour. Remember, though, that these exercises are too important to leave in a comfortable chair while your eyes are closed. When you were small, about five years of age you went to school, and one of the lessons you did was "sums". You did this sitting in a small chair at a small desk, with a teacher and a blackboard, an exercise book and a text book. The teacher drew something on the blackboard and you copied it and then did some more of the same out of your text book. At about half past three or four the bell rang and you put your text book and exercise book back in your desk, and the teacher cleaned the blackboard, and you went out to play. It was then, without realizing it, you did your sums. Every time you looked at a clock to tell the time you did sums. Every time you played a game with a score, you did sums. Every time you looked at a date or timetable you did sums. Every time you baked a cake you did sums. Every time you bought or sold anything you did sums. Sums were far too important to leave in a classroom in a little desk with a teacher and other children. Likewise the exercises in this book are far too important to leave in a comfortable chair while your eyes are closed and you are in an altered state. You must feel them, and do them, all the time without realizing it. Otherwise you won't get better.

EXERCISE 14. IDEO-MOTOR FINGER RESPONSES.

When you are talking to someone in a perfectly normal state of consciousness, and you are asking them a question to which they answer "yes", watch their head. Ask them another question to which they will answer "yes" and watch their head again. Most people answering "yes" to a question will not only say "yes", but at the same time they will nod their head. Ask them without telling them, "what did they do when they answered the question" and most of them won't have a clue what they did, showing that the nod of the head is an unconscious answer. The same is true of a negative answer when they shake the head.

While people are talking, even in a normal state of consciousness, two parts of their mind are listening, paying attention and answering. The conscious mind is answering by verbally saying "yes" or "no" but at the same time the unconscious mind is also answering by nodding or shaking the head. This nodding or shaking the head is called an ideo-motor response. It is a response from the unconscious mind. We often set this up deliberately so that we can explore the unconscious mind. If we are being affected by something which happened to us long ago, we must have a memory of it somewhere within us; if this were not the case, it would not be affecting us now. This memory, however, is often long since forgotten consciously, but it is still in the unconscious somewhere. We can explore the unconscious mind in an altered state by asking the unconscious to answer our questions by lifting a finger of one of our hands, say the index finger of the left hand, or often it is better to let the unconscious mind choose which finger it will use. It can use one finger for "yes" and another for "no", in this way we can ask it yes or no questions. You can even have an "I don't know" finger, and an "I don't want to answer" finger, but I feel having too many alternatives often confuses the answer. We are much less used to lying with our finger so we may well get a more honest answer this way. It is not, however, infallible and the finger can lie. So we just ask our unconscious mind if it will answer in this way and if it will, will it please lift a "yes" finger. One finger should rise. Establish a "no" finger in the same way and if you get a response both times you should be able to ask it some more questions that may help you to have more options. It is not so easy to do this by yourself but if it is first done with a therapist many patients can do it by themselves. The skill is often in knowing what to ask it, and what to do about it when you get an answer.

CHAPTER 4

From four years of age to the present day—Negative Conditioning —Third Line Trauma

The type of traumas inflicted upon us from four years of age onwards are generally between ourselves and the world and the people in it. Lack of loving contact is the most common one, along with a lack of understanding of our needs and total ignorance on the part of the inflictor of the devastating effect that simple negative statements may have had upon the recipient of those statements.

Humiliation
Humiliation is one of the more common traumas we experience and it frequently gives rise to some of our sharpest and most painful memories. Virtually everyone can recall with great clarity the details of their most humiliating experiences no matter how long ago these occurred. For instance, when I was four years of age and learning to write, my mother, whom I loved very much and who on the whole was very good to me, told me you could spell my first name, Geoffrey, in two ways. Not only could you spell it the way I have just spelt it, but you could also spell it Jeffrey. I believed her. When I was five, on my first day at school the headmaster gave all the new boys a pep talk and asked us all to write our names on a piece of paper. I wrote Jeffrey Graham. The following day he had us all together again, and he said there was only one boy in the school who couldn't spell his name, "Geoffrey Graham come out here to the front and let us see who you are." I wanted to cry, I tried to tell him but he

wouldn't listen, I wanted to kill him, but I could do none of those things, so I just hurt. When I got home I wanted to kick my mother but I loved her, and in any case she just said "you silly boy". I hated her, and hurt all the more. I have not been able to spell since for it hurt me too much to look at words to see how to spell them so I didn't look, and more times than not got them wrong. This reinforced my belief that I couldn't spell. I relived that trauma some time ago and I believe I could now learn to spell but I have got to a good age without being able to spell so it doesn't bother me so much, now that I have other priorities.

Funnily enough, very shortly after I had relived that trauma with a full release of the repressed emotions, who should come into my dental surgery with toothache as a casual patient, but the very same headmaster. I sat him in my chair and on examination found that a tooth had to come out. While I was giving him an injection of local anaesthetic I related to him the tale I have just told you, and he went as white as a sheet. I must have got over the hurt because I thought, "You poor sod, you just didn't know any better", and I felt sorry for him. I took his tooth out without any pain or bother, but you know he never came back.

An English master of mine, a few years later, used to get us to look at a picture or something and write a descriptive essay for the next day, as homework. One day he brought a bicycle pump into the class and took it to pieces. He said, "For your homework tonight I want you to write a descriptive essay on a bicycle pump". That night I thought 'to heck', and I wrote, 'I am a bicycle pump and my master has just taken me with his bicycle out for a run down to the seaside. As he is going along by the beach I fall off and roll down on to the sand where some children find me and they stick me on the top of a big sand castle by the sea. It's great fun, they are running all round me shouting and singing, but the tide is coming in and they are having to stand back. Now the sea is right round me and is getting higher up the castle towards me, and I am beginning to get frightened, and just as I am about to drown, my master sees me and wades out and plucks me from the waves and saves me from the sea. He puts me back on his bike and rides safely home with me'.

I handed it in the next morning, and when he had marked all the essays, he gave them all back except mine. He then said "listen to what this idiot Graham has written for a descriptive essay". He read it out to the class encouraging them to laugh at it all the way through. Again I could have killed him but I just hurt. I found my imagination just wouldn't work after that . . . not until I had relived it, expressing all the repressed emotions that I hadn't dared feel or express at the time. So you see how humiliation can reduce our options in life. For years I would shun situations where there was the slightest chance of anyone laughing at me, and of course it got reinforced. My release came when I took full responsibility for myself, and stopped blaming others.

On a similar note, I had a colleague, Alan, who asked me to help him with his shyness. He said he often went to professional meetings and at the end of such a meeting, during question time, he would have loved to have asked a question. However, he felt so embarrassed and frightened that he never dare stand up and ask his question. This annoyed him so much that when he got home after the meeting he would be furious with himself. His treatment was to create a Pavlovian conditioned response (see chapter 2) which would give him a resource which would help him in that particular circumstance. (See exercise 15 at the end of this chapter.) These two examples however, show how much the fear of humiliation can reduce our options in life and prevent us from enjoying the journey.

Strict upbringing, Religion, and Sexual attitudes

The strict, repressive upbringing which some children and young people undergo produces in them a range of behaviours displaying the extremes of anger fear and guilt. For example, a young woman of twenty-six was referred to me by her doctor as a "hopeless case". Janet was an acute anxiety-depressive, who was playing around with pot, speed, uppers, downers, alcohol and sex, and anything else she could get her hands on. Her parents and grandparents were very stiff, unfeeling, strict disciplinarians. Sex was a dirty word, never spoken about and strictly taboo. Janet had had a few not very serious attempts at overdosing, as she always told someone what she had done immediately after taking an overdose. She was terrified most of the time, unless she was "high" on what ever she could get hold of. I remember the first time Janet came to consult me she was fairly drunk.

No way could she cuddle either of her parents; they just weren't that sort. Nobody cuddled in her family. Everybody, including Janet herself, though she was a "bad" person. She was quite attractive and tried to flirt with me on the first visit.

I told her how sorry I was for her, and how awful it must be to be so frightened all the time, and have to put on such an act. The tears began to roll down her face, so I encouraged her to cry telling her it was O.K. to do that here. It was safe to cry here because it would show me how desperate she really was, without her having to put on an act for me. She sobbed even louder so I gently held her hand, encouraging her to cry. She said she had never in her life been able to do that with anyone. I just said "if she had, she wouldn't need to be here". She apologized for drinking before she came, and for trying to flirt, and said she realised for the first time she thought she would get the help she so desperately needed. I thanked her for her confidence in me, and said her genuine tears had helped me make up my mind that I could help her.

We worked together for about two and a half years over which time she had about twenty-five one hour sessions. I gradually built her confidence in herself, and helped her to see that what she was doing was wrong for herself, not for anyone else, and that she was responsible for how she was and felt. Janet began to see that her anxiety and depression were due to her behaviour and if she wanted to be comfortable she would have to change, and love herself. She saw that her behaviour was not deliberate but was the only thing she knew to do at the time; she also saw that, although unrecognized in the past she did have options and if she took some of these options she would be more comfortable. I encouraged Janet to review, in an altered state, her childhood and asked her to use whatever adult mind she had to comfort and love and understand her child mind. So it could grow up being loved. (See next chapter on becoming the parent you never had.)

Gradually Janet began to understand herself, and eventually to like herself. She stopped taking drugs and alcohol and playing around with everybody. She met a man and for the first time in her life fell in love. She then found it possible to love herself. Her anxiety and depression cleared, and she married her man, and has settled down and has two children whom she loves and cuddles.

In one of our sessions Janet relived being on holiday in Spain when she was a teenager. She was attracted to the boys but they were taboo, according to her mother. She dreamed one evening that an evil spirit had entered her room and she had swallowed it, and it was the evil spirit that was making her do all these "bad" things, and she was possessed. I got a Bible and crucifix and asked her to kiss them both, which she did, and I explained that she would not have been able to do that if she were possessed. It is amazing what guilt will make us do to feel better. It is also amazing how unreligious and unloving and non-understanding some religions can be. I find most forms of extreme behaviour, whether it be religion or whatever, seem to seriously restrict one's options in life, and make neurotic behaviour the commonest choice.

I used the Bible and crucifix because I belive that if you can prove a point by some simple action it is worth a thousand words. A look, a touch, a sigh, can convey great meaning. I often blow a raspberry with my hand and lips, when I feel sure a patient is swinging a line. It's amazing how effective it can be. I had a Christmas card from Janet some two years after the end of her treatment saying how well she still was, and how happy she was with her husband and two children. She had become a whole person, totally responsible for herself. Now four years later she is still living happily with her husband and family.

Forced Extreme Behaviour

When I was conducting a workshop-seminar in Dublin, Ireland, I was demonstrating a technique with the doctors on the workshop. One of the common complaints among doctors, resulting from a third line trauma, is an inability to relax and get to sleep easily. This complaint evolves from the unreasonably long hours a hospital junior doctor has to stay on duty. He has to stay awake and alert for so many hours that when his duty time is over he can't relax, or get to sleep easily. This eventually wears off for most of them, but a few remain unable to perform those two necessary functions in life for a long time afterwards.

I asked if anyone on the workshop had these difficulties, and as usual on such seminars, I had no difficulty in getting a volunteer. The charming doctor who volunteered said he "had the devil's own job getting to sleep". I asked if he had difficulty in sleeping, did he also feel tired during the day? His answer was a very firm "yes". I helped him into an altered state of consciousness, and asked him to go inside his mind and find that part of his mind that helped him to go to sleep. When the part of his mind that helped him was listening, paying attention, and was willing to negotiate, would it please lift his index finger of his right hand. (Ideo-motor finger control, see chapter 3.) His right index finger lifted fairly quickly. I them asked him to go inside his mind and find the part of his mind that helped him to stay awake. When that part was listening, paying attention, and willing to negotiate it could lift his left index finger. Fairly quickly his left index finger rose from his knee.

I now asked these two parts if we could negotiate and do a deal. If so, they could both return to his knee, which they both did, again, fairly quickly. I then said I would like to talk to the part controlling his right index finger, the part that helps him sleep. Would that part not make him tired during the day if his other part, the part that keeps him awake, would not keep him awake during the night? If that was O.K. his right index finger would rise, and it did. I then said I would talk to the part that keeps him awake, the part controlling his left index finger. Would that part not keep him awake during the night if the other part didn't make him tired during the day; if that was O.K. it could lift his left index finger. His left index finger rose high in the air. At this point I was going to ask a few more questions, but before I could, both his hands rose from his knees and came together, and his fingers clasped together. As I had wanted to ask some more questions I asked "what are your hands doing right now?" He answered in his lovely Irish brogue "sure they are shaking hands on the deal. It sounds like a good idea". I saw no point in asking any more questions.

(This technique forms the basis of Exercise 16—negotiating between parts. See the end of this chapter. And it also shows a part of the principle of reframing.) I hope it also demonstrates another aspect of third line trauma, in a light hearted manner.

Parental Arguments

Another very common third line trauma that is inflicted upon us is produced when our parents argue violently, either verbally or physically, and very often when the husband is drunk. Even if our parents argue when they think the children are not listening, most times the children are aware of it because it creates an atmosphere which children find very threatening. If you ever witness two parents arguing in front of the children, the children will often shout "Stop it, your hurting me", even if the argument has nothing to do with the children. They will often cower under a table, or behind a chair or door. If they witness an argument and are sent away to their room or boarding school that often makes it worse. Their imagination makes it fifty times worse; most times, if you ask them, they will tell you they would rather see how it ends.

I was treating a boy who bedwets while his two parents were present in my room with him. In an altered state, I told Simon that he would have to tell me the truth, and I then asked him what upset him most in life. He answered quite truthfully, "Mummy and Daddy fighting". I turned to look at his mother and father who were showing some embarrassment and said to both of them "What can you do to help your son's bedwetting?" They said "Nothing, we are just like that". Even when they know, they often can do very little about it. They seem trapped in their own neurosis, and unable to be aware of how much damage they are inflicting on their children. Very often it is again 'The sins of the fathers visiting the children'.

I told Simon he had two handicaps in his life. One was his parents, which he could do nothing about; he had just heard them say they couldn't help arguing. The other was his bedwetting, which was a self-inflicted handicap which he could either keep of give up, as it was serving a useless cause. The choice was his.

A very intelligent bank manager, who I shall call David was referred to me by his psychiatrist. David had a terrible motorway phobia which was now affecting him even when he got in his car to drive anywhere. He was in his forties and single, with no previous history of any psychiatric illness. He admitted some difficulty in settling arguments at his bank between the staff, which was one of his functions as manager. He couldn't cuddle either of his parents, they were not that sort. His parents had had quite violent verbal arguments when he was small, and his mother had always threatened to leave his father at the end of the row. While he hid under the table during these rows he often wished he were dead, or that his parents had not had him. (The 'blame game'.) Now that he had grown up he realised that his parents were 'just like that,' and anyway they were settling down a little in their old age.

David's phobia had first manifested itself when he was driving his car on a motorway to visit his parents. Just prior to his driving to his old home he had had a row with his fiancée. She had told him she was going off with someone else. Feeling quite upset, David set off down the motorway to visit home. Fairly soon after he got on to the motorway, his legs seemed to turn to jelly and he had quite a job stopping the car on the hard shoulder. He got out to have a walk, his body shaking all over. It was quite some time before David dared to return to his car and drive it off the motorway. He did this with some difficulty, which he found strange because he was an advanced motorist and had passed his advanced motoring test to prove it. The next time he went to get in his car he felt very apprehensive and had to have valium and a glass of whisky before he could drive. His fear gradually got worse until he couldn't drive anywhere without being pretty well doped up.

David realised he had probably been lucky that he had not married his fiancée before she had left him, and he felt he had got over that now, but his phobia was getting steadily worse. It took about three visits to get this information out of him, and with some relaxing exercises he was still no better.

After another session with still no progress I decided we should try something else. In an altered state I had him relive the first time he felt frightened on the motorway and I had him relate to me every feeling he was experiencing. He began to get more and more agitated and cried "I wish I was dead". He was going to visit his mother and father. He had just had a big argument with his lady friend. His conditioned response to arguments from his childhood was 'I wish I was dead,' especially when his mother threatened to leave his father. His fiancée had just left him for someone else. What else could he feel under the circumstances with such conditioning? There was enough of his adult mind left to stop him from killing himself by driving into something at speed, though the idea frightened the living daylight out of him and, incidentally, stopped him from doing it by rendering him unable to drive the car. He had now, however, anchored driving with fear and killing himself, in his unconscious mind, so it had to continue to make it impossible for him to do that by making him incapable of driving. I often wonder what might have happened if someone had been able to hypnotise him and, with symptom removal, got rid of his phobia without removing the anchor feeling of wanting to kill himself.

I reframed his behaviour towards arguments, and his feelings towards women, and made him more and more aware of his real needs and desires and left his fear of driving alone. After one of our sessions he said I thought you would like to know that I got engaged to be married last weekend. It was the end of the morning for me and I had two hours before my next patient. I went outside with him and asked him to get into my car. I took him to the nearest motorway and drove very fast, down to the next turn off. When we were off the motorway I told him to change places with me and drive my car back up the motorway to where we had come from. He did this without any bother and at quite a speed. When we stopped back at my consulting rooms he looked at me and asked me how I knew he would be able to drive alright. I told him "you don't want to kill yourself any more". David got married and introduced me to his wife and he has been able to drive his car ever since.

Sibling Rivalry for Love and Attention
Another very common third line trauma results from the rivalry that goes on between children in the family for love from parents. As mentioned in the previous chapter the elder child often develops asthma, or starts bedwetting when the next child is born. This often is made worse when the older child has reached school age. Sending them off to school is seen as just another rejection, leaving the younger child a clear field to get all the love. If this is felt by the child going to school they often don't do as well as they might have done at school, and the school gets the blame, once again playing the 'blame game'. Sometimes the elder child just becomes 'difficult', agressive or rude. The parents, trying to correct this 'difficult' nature, just confirm they prefer the younger child, and the elder one is left to hurt by their own behaviour, and move further away from their real needs, having in the end to deny those needs.

It is a natural desire for many parents to hope for one of each sex if they have two children. I myself am a second son. My parents decided to try once again after me and they hit the jackpot and got a daughter. I remember clearly, even now after fifty years, thinking after my sister was born, 'What is going to happen to me now'? I thought my elder brother seemed to be so much cleverer than me (naturally as he was older, he was). My younger sister seemed to give my parents so much joy that I didn't seem to be able to give them, so I just hurt. I had to prove myself over and over again, and go on proving myself, long after it was necessary or reasonable. Most of this behaviour was unconscious at the time, and I only realised it during one of my personal growth sessions.

This enabled me to take responsibility for myself and only compete with myself after that, thus giving me release from the need of having to prove myself. I hope this illustrates what a difficult position being a second son followed by a daughter, or second daughter followed by a son can be. It generally leaves the middle one having to prove themselves quite unreasonably, and very often they are not aware of it consciously.

With large families it is often very difficult for the first one. Each time another child is born they feel it as another rejection of them and begin to think 'What is the matter with me?' They often end up needing repeated confirmation that they are lovable, but are also often unable to accept that love. This depends on how hurt this process has made them feel. That which hurt me when I was small is far too hurtful for me to accept now. (See Bill in chapter 3.) Real love seems to smother them, so they end up flirting madly to get this confirmation that they are lovable, until the relationship gets serious, only to break it off, and move on to the next affair. This is an unconscious reaction which reinforces the feeling of there being 'something wrong with them' which makes the next affair all the more important to confirm they are lovable, and confirms to them they don't know what love is.

We should perhaps look at the case of the 'only child' and try to see what effect that may have. Often the 'only child' has to grow up too quickly when it is really still a child. It forms adult thoughts with childish concepts, consequently when it becomes adult many of its concepts remain childish.

I hope this section on sibling rivalry shows you how the position in the family is important, how it can hurt, and how it may be driving you quite unconsciously to behaviours that you find difficult to understand. These behaviours are often very restrictive and annoying to the person having them and only reinforces the hurt.

Reactive Depression

Reactive depression is a reaction to a disaster, family tragedy, or individual misfortune, which goes on long after normal grief, or sorrow, should have ended. The most common causes include a broken love affair, the failure of an ambition, the leaving home of adored children or child, or the death of a loved one. It is right and proper that if you should lose a loved one, you should feel sad and weepy for a time, but if that time goes on and on for years and years, then it becomes pathological. There are three common causes of this pathological depression. One is an over-indulgence in self pity, often associated with an over-dependence on the lost one, or thing. The second is to relieve a guilt feeling, that you weren't as good to the lost one, or thing, as you should have been. A third reason, which is getting more common now, is when the person doesn't feel the grief at the time of the loss. This is often due to too may tranquilizers being prescribed immediately after the loss. (For treatment see exercise 17, at the end of this Chapter.)

Patients suffering from third line traumas tend to be highly intellectualized individuals. They have much less control of their body, and are less co-ordinated. They have either less sexdrive or a highly symbolized sexual activity. They tend to relate to ideas or numbers rather than being able to relate in an emotional way to other human beings. They often end up as accountants, doctors, engineers or teachers.

Many people have first, second and third line traumas all on top of each other, each one reinforcing the other. It is often impossible for these people not to inflict pain on their children. 'THE SINS OF THE FATHERS VISIT THE CHILDREN UNTIL THE SEVENTH GENERATION'.

If you know which symptoms are produced by which line you can often save time in trying to find the cause of the behaviour by having a good idea when the original trauma occurred, (which line [time] imprinted or conditioned that behaviour?) A learnt behaviour can lie dormant for years before something triggers it off, and reinforces it.

EXERCISE 15. CREATING NEW RESOURCES FROM OLD.

In the case of my colleague, Alan, who was frightened to get up and ask a question at a professional meeting for fear of humiliation, I had him think of a time in the past when he wanted to show off, or was very brave. He had some diffi-

FOUR YEARS OF AGE TO THE PRESENT DAY 47

culty in remembering an occasion, but eventually told me his mother reminded him of when they used to go to the beach. The particular beach they went to had a wall running along the edge. When Alan was small he would run along the wall and when he reached a high part, he would shout, "Mummy, Mummy look at me" and then jump onto the sand. The resource he was feeling at the time of shouting to his mummy had to be, "Aren't I clever?, I want you to see how clever I am and tell me". Wouldn't that be a good resource to feel at a meeting if he wanted to ask a question, and wouldn't it help him to overcome his fear if he could feel it?

I had Alan in an altered state review that scene on the beach while he shouted "Mummy! Mummy! look at me". While he was feeling as much of that scene as he could he was to rub his thumb over the tips of his fourth, middle and index fingers. The rubbing of his fingertips with his thumb is equivalent to Pavlov's bell. Feeling the scene is equivalent to Pavlov's feeding the dogs, so by doing that for about two to three minutes at a time, about five times a day, for twenty days he was creating a simple Pavlovian conditioned reflex of feeling, "Aren't I clever?, I want you to see how clever I am", to rubbing his fingertips. After that time he would be able to feel "Aren't I clever?, I want you to see how clever I am", by just rubbing his fingertips together. I feel it is a nice concept of having resources at your fingertips. So the next time he was at a meeting, and he wanted to ask a question, after he had created the reflex, all he had to do was to rub his fingertips together, and get up and ask away.

If you are afraid to do something then create a conditioned reflex to feeling brave from a time when you were actually brave, or stood up for someone or something. You can create a feeling of confidence from a time when you were happy and confident. All you need is a time in the past when you had a resource that would be useful now in the behaviour you would like to change, create the reflex, and go ahead with the new feeling from the past.

EXERCISE 16.   NEGOTIATING BETWEEN THE PARTS.
When there are two functions, both of which are necessary

(but at different times) and these are interfering with each other, it is possible to help the situation and behaviour by negotiating between the two parts of the mind responsible for those two functions. See the example above, in sleeping and being awake. Another example is in concentration while working and relaxing afterwards, or learning to switch off.

Many people who have very demanding, busy, and exacting jobs find great difficulty in switching off, at weekends or evenings, without some form of drug etc. Commonly the drug thought to be the lesser of the evils is alcohol. Perhaps this is why there are so many alcoholics in the professions. Wouldn't it be much better to learn to switch off with our minds instead of alcohol, or whatever? To do that, all that is necessary is to enter an altered state of consciousness and go inside the mind and find the respective parts responsible first for concentration, then for relaxation. Thank both parts for their respective functions. Ask each to listen, pay attention, and be willing to negotiate. Set up an ideo-motor response for both parts in one or another of each index finger (as in text of chapter 4). Negotiate first with one part then with the other and ask each to respond as in text of chapter 4. Having got a response from each, ask them to confirm their willingness to begin to help you in this new negotiated way, from right now, by coming together and touching, as a token of shaking hands on the deal, as our wonderful Irish friend put it. I always use what people come up with if it is a good idea.

EXERCISE 17.   FOR REACTIVE DEPRESSION.
First of all it is necessary to find out what is causing the depression, or which of the three reasons, mentioned in the text, is responsible for the negative feelings. The first question is "did you cry and feel really bad at the time?" If not, you possibly haven't felt it all, and need to. The second question is "do you miss not having the person around and will nothing, or no one, ever be able to replace your need for them?" If the answer is yes to both those questions then you have too great a dependence on someone else and need to become your own parent. The third question is "do you feel bad that they are no longer here and you won't ever be able to

tell them how much you loved them?" If the answer is yes, you are suffering from guilt. You may be suffering from one, two, or all three of these reasons.

If you haven't felt the grief then it is probably better to find a therapist to help you to do that by talking about it openly, while the therapist encourages you to feel what you are talking about, and at the same time provides the necessary support while you are doing so. Entering an altered state will often facilitate the release of repressed feelings, or hyperventilating will do the same. Either of these techniques should be done with the support of a good therapist, in case you get into a feeling that you can't handle on your own.

If you are overdependent on the lost one, you need to become the parent you never had. It may be the lost one is not your parent, but overdependence is always a child-parent relationship, and you are using a parent substitute. Remember the purpose of life is to mature and become responsible for yourself. Most of the exercises in this book are designed to help you become the parent you never had, and mature, and become responsible for yourself.

It may be useful for you to remember that the good experiences you had with the lost one can't be taken away from you by their not being here. An experience is an experience that you have had, and can't be taken away, because you have already had it. It is your experience for the rest of your life. You may not be able to repeat the experience, but that which you have had can't be taken away from you. I am sure your loved one would like to live on in your memory as a good experience, and not as a sad feeling. In exactly the same way, I'm sure when you go, you would like your loved ones to remember you with the good experiences you have had together, and not with bad feelings.

If you feel bad, and guilty, because you never told your lost one how much you really loved them, remember that to feel bad about them when they have gone is like rubbing salt into the wound. You can show them how much you really love them by feeling really good about the good things about them, and using those good things to sustain you for the rest of your life. So tell yourself all the good things you know about your lost one, in an altered state, and feel really good that you had such a good store of good experiences with them. This way you can show the world how much you loved them.

CHAPTER 5

Becoming your own Parent

During the first nine months of your life, while you are in the womb, the womb and cord are your providers. They give you a world to live in, that is, hopefully, safe and secure. They supply every need via the cord without you having to ask for anything. When you get out, however, the cord is cut, your world takes on a new dimension. Your providers become legion. Initially your parents are your providers, but no parent can provide everything for you, all the time without you having to ask for it. Therefore the purpose of life is to become your own parent and provider. The only truly happy people are those who succeed in this quest. The process of maturation is to become your own provider, to become responsible for self, and capable of living with yourself. When you are capable of living with yourself, it is then safe to choose who you will share your life with, without becoming too dependent on them. You can only love someone properly, when you learn to love yourself; you can't give to someone else what you haven't got for yourself.

Many people, for the reasons outlined in the previous three chapters, don't reach adult maturity, even when they are chronologically old enough to do so. The only way they can mature is for them to become the parent they didn't have.

In the following two examples I demonstrate the ways in which childhood traumas manifest themselves in later life. In the first of these cases, I shall refer to the subject as John.

John is a highly qualified and well respected professional in middle age. He seems to be rational, secure and well adjusted. John is a very dear friend who helps me organise some of the workshops that I run in the U.S.A. When I work on volunteers with problems, by helping them to comfort 'their child in themselves', he always feels weepy. He told me one evening when we had finished a workshop that my methods of treatment really got to him. His own childhood had been very difficult and painful. John's father had been a circuit judge, and each evening when he came home he had passed judgement on his son John. The judgement was always damning, and the punishment often physical. John was always in trouble, and never shown any physical love, consequently when his children were born and he held them, he could not feel any love for them, try as he may. He said "they might as well have been bundles of washing for all I could feel". It is only when they had grown up a little that he could feel anything for them, and only on an intellectual level. He had great difficulty in showing any loving feelings as he didn't recognise that feeling in himself. I am sure he admired his own intelligence, but felt no love for himself. If ever the love he had from his wife was threatened, he would get very possessive and angry.

I asked him to close his eyes and access one of the childhood scenes where his father was being aggressive towards him and, as much as he could, to feel how upset his 'child mind' was. Watching his 'child mind' feeling hurt, he was to take his 'adult mind' and comfort his 'child', telling his 'child' that he would love him, and respect him, so that he never need feel hurt again about that scene. John protested that he couldn't love his 'child' as his 'child' had been so bad. This 'bad' feeling was a conditioned response to always being told he was no good and never would be any use to anyone. I said to him he had some options. He could go on feeling upset and restricted in the way he felt, or could find a way to love and help his 'child' to grow up in a loving atmosphere. A couple of days later he said "blast it I am going to find a way to love my 'child' ".

That was during my last visit to the United States. I do not know whether John acted upon his decision to love his 'child self'. However, I do know that he can only increase his options and change his feelings if he makes a determined effort to overcome the effect of his deep seated trauma. The weepiness he was experiencing, when I was working with other people, was a sure sign of the dynamic inner process he was undergoing. Only a dynamic process would be able to affect him so dramatically. If he can still cry about it, it is still affecting him.

It is important to realise that we are all constantly developing and it is often impossible to say how far we have travelled along the road towards becoming our own parents, I am sure we only make a start on that journey when we start to love ourselves, as our 'child' selves.

A patient, Frank, came for help because he always felt tired, and couldn't concentrate on anything for more than a few seconds. He told me that, when he was a child, whenever he was doing anything his father would come up to him and say, "That's no good! you are useless, you will never be able to do anything right". Being told he was no good was reinforced over and over again on thousands of occasions until he began to believe it. The only way he could defeat his father was to be useless. This seemed to get his father mad, so by being useless he won. The trouble is though, his father has been dead for years, and Frank is still winning by losing. He cannot do anything else; he has no options.

I started by reminding him of the marathon he won all by himself. Then, as he had won that marathon, he had just as much right as any other person to be here. Just as much as his father. I had him do all the exercises at the end of chapter 1, as an introduction to believing in himself, and a start to becoming his own parent.

I had Frank review his childhood in an altered state to see how much his father's cruelty had hurt him, making a note of the occasions he felt most hurt. I asked him what he felt for his father. He replied that he hated him. So I asked what sort of father did he think he was. He said he was useless. So I asked him, 'Who was the one that was useless, your father or yourself?".

Frank answered "My father".

"Yes he was a pretty useless father wasn't he?"

"He certainly was".

"Why then do you still need to win, and beat him, by losing?"

"I don't".
"What would you do if you had a son in the circumstances where your father told you, you were useless?"
"I would help him to do it himself. My father never let me do anything. He always said I couldn't do it, so he used to push me out of the way and do it himself. I would show my son, he could do it. And I would show him I loved him".
"How would you do that?"
"I would cuddle him, and talk to him nicely, and show him that I cared for him".
"Do you think he would feel much more loved, than you do?"
"Yes".
"Would he want to win by failing?'
"Certainly not! he wouldn't need to, would he?" Frank replied.
"No! Do you?"
"No!"
"Good".

EXERCISE 18.   Still in an altered state of consciousness I asked Frank to review the first of the hurtful episodes he had spoken about earlier, as if it were a film. While he was watching himself as a child, (his 'child's mind'), he was to go to his "child self", and tell that little boy that he loved him. That he understands him. That he will help him to grow up. That his 'child self' need never feel so alone or hurt again. That he can be anything he really wants, and he doesn't need to fail to win because he (his 'adult mind') will help his 'child self'. We then went through each of the traumas Frank had remembered in the altered state, asking his 'adult mind' to comfort and encourage the child Frank in each case as above. When we finished, we asked his unconscious mind to indicate with an ideo-motor finger response if there were any more occasions he felt alone, or afraid, hurt and unloved. Of course, there were others which we had to work through. I then worked on reframing Frank's defences, by showing him that there were much better ways to defend himself as an adult, than losing, and it would be much easier if he was able to concentrate for as long as necessary. I told him he could really beat his father by being successful. (End of Exercise 18.)

Slowly Frank's concentration improved and he felt less tired. He was able to work on a number of the traumas by himself, each time being the ideal parent that the boy Frank didn't have. He was able to see the reasons for his behaviour much more clearly, which gave him more options. Occasionally he still gets a feeling he doesn't understand so he returns for a session and we sort it out, and he takes over control for himself again.

I hope the example of treatment in Frank's case shows you how to become your own parent in the case of third line trauma.

The above technique is also how I worked with Janet, whose strict upbringing had caused her great pain, (see previous chapter). In her case, while she was in that altered state we call hypnosis, I had her fantasize she was holding the little girl Janet on her knee. She actually put her arms round her imagined younger self and cuddled her while she was telling her she loved and respected her. I find this physical action of holding your imagined self, while you are telling your younger self that you love and respect them, is very useful both in helping you to feel that you do love your younger self, and in creating the circumstances whereby you can begin to be able to love yourself as an adult. You start by loving your younger self and in doing so find that you can love your adult self. This is a very necessary part of the treatment (see the end of the first paragraph in this chapter).

For second line traumas (traumas that occurred from a few hours after birth to six year of age. Traumas that generally arise from the need for attention which you did not get.) the process of becoming your own parent is similar to the technique above.

EXERCISE 19.   In the hypnotic state, first find out from your unconscious mind what attention you needed and didn't get, then have yourself fantasize giving yourself that attention while you are holding your younger self. At the same time reassure your younger self that they need never feel so alone or afraid again because you will give them all the attention they need to grow up in a safe, secure and loving environment. Reassure your younger self that they needn't resort to desperate means (the symptoms produced to get attention by your 'child self'), or even the neurotic behaviour that they are making you carry out now, to get attention because you (the adult you) will help them (the child you) to find more adult ways of getting attention. Or better still to find ways of coping without needing attention (becoming responsible for self, the process of maturing, and the purpose of life). (End of exercise 19.)

First line traumas generally arise from a misunderstanding of what is happening at birth. This is brought about by the very traumatic nature of the birth itself in most births, and the totally unknown magnitude of the experience of birth to the birthing child. Sometimes these traumas are due to the ignorance of those delivering the baby and their total lack of understanding of the baby's needs at birth. The way to become the parent you never had, in the case of 'birth trauma' patients is to get them to view their situation from a position one step removed from the 'action'. This process, known as dissociation, is designed to protect the patient from the full force of the pain of a relived trauma. The method can be seen in the following examples.

In the case of Tom, the breech birth example in chapter 2, it was essential to have him dissociate his mind from his body, because if you tried to regress him, using hypnosis, to his birth, his body had such a strong memory of the very traumatic nature of the birth that he would automatically begin to abreact and feel the pain of the birth. This made it impossible for him to take his adult mind and comfort his birthing self because his birthing self took over completely and left no room for any adult mind. (See the end of the previous paragraph.)

EXERCISE 20. In Tom's case, I had him enter the state of hypnosis (altered state of consciousness), and while relaxing, create an image of himself in a cinema, first of all with the screen blank. While he was looking at the blank screen, he was to take his mind to the row behind his body, thus watching his body in the row in front watching the screen. This way he couldn't feel his body in the row in front. He was then to watch himself, in the row in front, watching a film of his birth on the screen. With his mind he was to see his 'baby self' stuck, with his legs out, and everybody trying to get his head out safely. He was to take his mind to the screen, leaving his body back in the cinema watching his mind talking to his 'baby self'. His mind was to tell his 'baby self' that he knew his 'baby self' would get out safely because his mind was his 'baby self' from the future. His mind was also to tell his 'baby self' that everybody involved wanted to help him get out safely and no one wanted to hurt him, let alone pull his head off. His mind was to tell his 'baby self' that his mother wanted him alive and well and she loved him very much, but during the birth she couldn't tell him that, so Tom must now tell him. His 'adult' mind was to use all its power of persuasion to convince his 'baby self' that all these things were true, and to help his 'baby self' get out feeling safe, loved and wanted. When his 'baby self' had got out believing these things, he was to tell it he loved it and then go back to the row behind his body in the cinema. He was then to go back into his body seeing his 'baby self' 'out', safe, and feeling loved by everybody. He was to repeat this exercise until he felt his 'baby self' believed him. It took quite a time before this happened, but when it did he no longer had any fear of having his head knocked off in places with people serving behind counters. (End of exercise 20.)

EXERCISE 21. In the case of migraine, have the patient dissociate their mind from their body and watch a film of their birth with their head stuck. Have their mind tell their 'baby self' that by decreasing their intra-cranial pressure they made it possible for them to get their head out more easily but they never need do that again unless they are being actually reborn. When they are 'out' have their mind tell their 'baby self' that the reflation helped them to restore the shape of their head, but they never need do that again especially when their cranial bones are fully united. Tell them that everyone loves them including yourself and they are wanted and no one was trying to get rid of them, or wipe them out. Tell them you will show them much more mature ways of dealing with stress (see the next chapter).

EXERCISE 22. Patients suffering from depression should see themselves stuck, in the birth canal, generally with the head through the arch and their shoulders stuck, unable to go forwards or backwards. Have their 'adult minds' tell their 'baby self' that the only defence in this situation is to stop feeling but that their 'adult mind' knows that they will get 'out' safely because their 'adult mind' is their 'baby self' from the future. Reassure them that everybody wants them 'out' and safe, and everybody loves them. Have their 'adult mind' see their 'baby self' get 'out' and persuade the 'baby self' that it is both safe and necessary to feel again. It is especially necessary to feel that they are 'out' and it is no longer unsafe to feel. In the future there will be much better defences, to situations in which they may feel stuck, than not feeling. To 'not feel' in future situations will just ensure that they are unable to do anything about the unpleasant positions they may find themselves in. Have them repeat this exercise until they begin to feel again, and their depression begins to lift. Then teach them new defences to stress. (See next chapter.)

EXERCISE 23. With patients suffering from Anorexia Nervosa, have them see themselves struggling to get 'out' and in the struggle getting the cord entangled. Have their adult mind see and persuade their 'baby self', that it is nobody's fault especially their 'friend and provider', the cord, or their mother. In any case have their 'baby mind' see that they do get 'out' safely and that in future they have no cause to reject the 'provider' (sustenance for themselves in the form of food) or 'mother' or blame either of them. They do not need to reject mother by killing themselves by not eating, as she was not guilty of trying to kill them. They do not need to be afraid of growing up and taking responsibility because they did ask to be here by winning a marathon and the purpose of being here is to mature. It is no use fighting the purpose of life because you can't win. If you die you just have to do it all over again so you may as well find a way of enjoying the journey and making it to that higher plane this time round. Have them repeat this exercise until they can respond to all the other treatment, some of which is described in chapter 2. This exercise will give them the parent (the need to mature and become responsible) they thought quite wrongly they didn't have at birth. (End of exercise 23.)

With all these exercises in this chapter if you have to use dissociation it is essential that the patient is capable of producing this hypnotic phenomenon. It is fortunately easy to test the patient's ability to dissociate by using Spiegel's Hypnotic Induction Profile test which only takes about five minutes to assess the patient's capabilities.

If you have a patient you find can't look you comfortably in the eyes, while you are talking to them, ask them if they have difficulty in doing that. If they do have difficulty most other people will reject them because the other people will not be able to trust them, and possibly think they are a little 'shifty'. The most likely cause of this difficulty is that the patient never bonded with their parent immediately following the birth. To establish a bond you can rebirth the patient and bond with them yourself, or get the patient to bond with themselves, or better still use both these options.

EXERCISE 24. To bond with yourself enter the hypnotic state and watch a film of yourself being born. Immediately you are born ('out') take your 'adult mind' to your 'baby self' and hold your 'baby self' lovingly while your 'adult mind' looks lovingly into your 'baby self's' eyes. When you can see that loving look returned by your 'baby self' the bond has been established and the patient will find it much easier to look people in the eyes without feeling uncomfortable. Repeat this exercise until you have no difficulty in looking people straight in the eyes.

I hope you can now see the importance of becoming the parent you never had and the ways of doing that.

CHAPTER 6
Stress

In chapter 2, I have talked about the stresses of birth and how they imprint behaviour. Then in chapter 3, we looked at the period from a few hours after birth to six years of age: how the stress of needing attention and not getting it creates different imprinted and conditioned behaviours. We then looked at the period in our life from four years of age to the present day, in chapter 4. We considered some of the things that may happen to us during that period of time which could condition our behaviour.

We all talk about stress and how the modern way of life has created an enormous increase in the effects of stress so let us now look at what stress is. To quote R. R. Tilleard-Cole in his book, 'The Fundamentals of Psychological Medicine', **'The purpose of a nervous system is the provision of a feedback mechanism such that an input stimulus can alter the response of the whole organism'**. This corresponds to our imprinted and conditioned responses.

'The input stimulus comes not only from within the body to provide internal homeostasis.' (learned behaviour), **but also from the external environment.** (Those things we have been looking at in chapters 2, 3 and 4.) Tilleard-Cole then goes on to say **'Normal life can only exist if the response is appropriate to the input stimulus.'** At those times we have looked at, the response we made was generally the only option we had, and therefore was appropriate. If that behaviour becomes learned and repeated at later times (when) the circumstances may be totally different then the responses may be wholly inappropriate.

'STRESS is those factors, both in the environment and in

the feedback mechanism, which results in inappropriate responses, leading to an increase of the problem'. In other words STRESS is those sort of things we have been looking at in chapters 2, 3 and 4, together with our learned responses which because of the change of circumstances not only don't help the problem but make it worse. The way we are trying to help the problem becomes the problem.

'These factors cause an increase of either physical or mental tension or both, and a movement even further removed from homeostasis' or in other words our attempt to solve the problem in many cases has made it worse, or has even become the problem itself. It becomes the problem itself when there is a prolonging of the behaviour after the stimulus has long since been removed. This is a reasonably common occurrence with learned behaviours, and is generally due to our inability to get rid of the tension produced by the stress. Our system just keeps building up more and more tension until we can take no more, then it leaks out in neurotic behaviour.

THE STIMULUS RESPONSE DIAGRAM

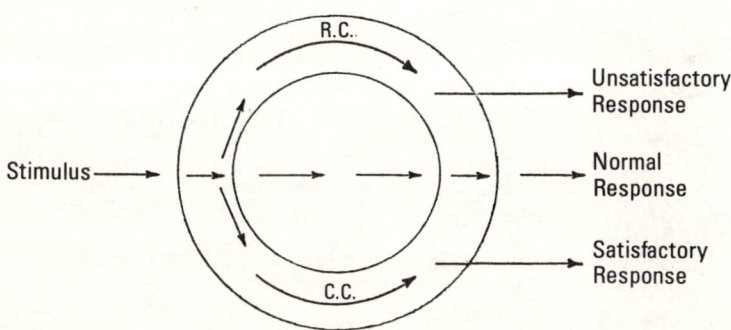

R.C. = REVERBERATING CIRCUIT OF LEARNED BEHAVIOUR.

C.C. = CORRECTING CIRCUIT USED IN REFRAMED BEHAVIOUR.

The increase in physical or mental tension, or both, often remains in our system long after the event has passed. The main problem is that many people either don't recognize the symptoms of that stress, or don't have enough ways of getting rid of it. The tension just builds up in our system until our system breaks down and we become ill.

What evidence is there that the sequence of events described in the above statement actually happens? Two people called Holmes, and Rahe, working for the United States Navy, were asked if it was possible to tell who might be ill during the next six months of their lives. The Navy wanted to know if it were possible to predict the likely sickness patterns of personnel serving in an atomic submarine that may be submerged under the icecap for a long period of time. If the officers or men on such missions were to fall ill it would be inconvenient at the very least: it might even threaten the success of the mission or the safety of the vessel.

Holmes and Rahe researched the factors which might lead to an increase in sickness levels. They found that some illness is caused by the stress of adjusting to those changes most of us encounter at some stage in our lives. They also found that certain changes were more likely to cause illness than others and were therefore able to compile a scale of the stress associated with each change of personal circumstance. (See scale they drew up below.)

HOLMES AND RAHE.

STRESS OF ADJUSTING TO CHANGE

DEATH OF HUSBAND OR WIFE	100
DIVORCE	73
MARITAL SEPARATIONS	65
DEATH OF CLOSE MEMBER OF FAMILY	63
JAIL SENTENCE	63
ILLNESS OR INJURY	53
MARRIAGE	50
LOSS OF JOB	47
RETIREMENT	45
HEALTH PROBLEM OF FAMILY	44
PREGNANCY	40
SEX PROBLEM	39
MAJOR CHANGES AT WORK	39
CHANGE OF FINANCIAL STATUS	38
DEATH OF A CLOSE FRIEND	37

INCREASE IN MARITAL ARGUMENTS	35
LARGE MORTGAGE TAKEN ON	31
CHILD LEAVES HOME	29
IN-LAW PROBLEMS	29
MAJOR PERSONAL ACHIEVEMENT	28
WIFE STOPS, OR STARTS WORK	26
STARTING/LEAVING EDUCATION	26
CHANGE IN LIVING CONDITIONS	25
TROUBLE WITH EMPLOYER	23
CHANGE IN RESIDENCE	20
CHANGE IN RECREATION	19
SMALL MORTGAGE/BANK LOAN	17
CHANGE IN SLEEPING HABITS	16
CHANGE IN FAMILY GET TOGETHER	15
CHANGE IN EATING HABITS	15
CHRISTMAS	12
MINOR VIOLATION OF THE LAW	11

People were given the above list and asked, 'Have any of the things in this list happened to you during the last year? If they have please tick'. Afterwards the number of ticks with their rating numbers were added up and it was found that people with a score of over 160 have a high probability of suffering from a breakdown in health during the next six months. This was tested with different cultures and classes and found to be reasonably consistent. Subsequently other scales of a similar nature have been drawn up and tested and all show similar results. I believe this shows quite conclusively that stress builds up in our system and leads to breakdown and illness.

Statistics from the medical profession in both the U.K. and the U.S.A. show that up to seventy percent of all patients currently being treated by doctors in General Practice are suffering from conditions which have their origins in unrelieved stress. The common treatments in General Practice for this stress are tranquillisers or anti-depressant drugs. None of these drugs are specific for any of the things we have looked at in chapters 2, 3 or 4. All of these drugs have side effects that are detrimental to the patients health. THE MOST POWERFUL AND YET MOST NEGLECTED THERAPEUTIC TOOL IS THE HUMAN MIND.

64 HOW TO BECOME THE PARENT YOU NEVER HAD

ENVIRONMENTAL CONDITIONS	MENTAL DATA	SYSTEM BUILDUP	

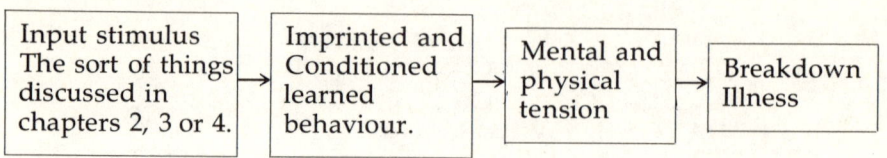

What are the illnesses already recognised as having stress at their foundation?

1. Hypertension—High blood pressure.
2. Coronary thrombosis.
3. Migraine.
4. Hay fever, and allergies. (See next chapter.)
5. Asthma.
6. Pruritus—Intense itching.
7. Peptic ulcers.
8. Constipation.
9. Colitis.
10. Rhematoid Arthritis.
11. Menstrual difficulties.
12. Nervous dyspepsia—Flatulence and indigestion.
13. Hyperthyroidism—over active thyroid gland.
14. Diabetes Mellitus.
15. Skin disorders.
16. Tuberculosis.
17. Depression.

And probably many others.

How do we recognise this build up of tension in our systems, preferably before we get ill?

Physical Symtoms of Stress

1. Lack of appetite.
2. Craving for food when under pressure.
3. Frequent indigestion or heartburn.

4. Constipation or Diarrhoea.
5. Insomnia.
6. Constant tiredness.
7. Tendency to sweat for no good reason.
8. Nervous tics.
9. Nail biting.
10. Headaches.
11. Cramps and muscle spasms.
12. Nausea.
13. Breathlessness without exertion.
14. Fainting spells.
15. Frequent crying or desire to cry, without conscious reason.
16. Impotency or frigidity, very often not admitted because of imagined shame.
17. Inability to sit still without fidgeting.
18. High blood pressure.

So if we find we are showing a few of the above physical symtoms we should start doing some of the things that lower tension. (See later in this chapter.)

Mental Symptoms of Stress

1. 'Constant irritability with people'. This happens even with people who would normally get on well with others.
2. 'Feeling of being unable to cope'. With life, your job, your husband or wife, your family, or anything that you would normally be able to cope with.
3. 'Lack of interest in life'. The 'I didn't ask to be here' people. Remind them that they won a marathon to be here, so they DID ask to be here.
4. 'Constant, or recurrent fear of disease'. (the cancer phobic patient, see chapter 3.) These people generally have an unconscious feeling of guilt due to first and second line trauma.
5. 'A feeling of being a failure'. (See chapter 5, 'Frank'.) This feeling is typical of third line trauma patients who have been conditioned by their parents who constantly told them they should do better.

6. 'A feeling of being bad or of self hatred'. (See 'Janet', chapter 4.) Also generally due to third line trauma caused by over strict upbringing, but can be due to first line (see next chapter).

7. 'Difficulty in making decisions'. This is generally due to having to get love from parents by always doing what they want and stifling what you feel you would like to do. (See paragraph before 'Think Feel' theory in chapter 2).

8. 'A feeling of ugliness'. One of my dental patients once asked me to crown her six front teeth because, she said, they made her ugly. Her teeth were perfectly sound and not mal-positioned. In fact there was nothing wrong with her teeth at all. She begged me, and said she would pay anything to have them done. I talked to her for a while and it became obvious she was suffering from stress. We left the dental consulting room and I 'put on my other hat' when we went in to the psychotherapy room. With a few sessions of psychotherapy and instruction in tension release she became quite happy with her front teeth, and had more options in her life. I shudder to think what could have happened if some unscrupulous person had tried to crown her teeth for the money offered. I can see no way she would have ended up satisfied with them, as there was nothing wrong with them in the first place.

9. 'Loss of interest in other people'. People who just want to be left alone.

10. 'Awareness of suppressed rage or anger'. The person who feels they are about to blow their top any minute now, for no apparent reason.

11. 'Inability to show true feelings'. Generally due to first or second line trauma.

12. 'A feeling of being the target of other people's animosity'. A patient once consulted me because he believed everybody thought he was a homosexual. He said he wasn't. I asked him if anyone had ever actually accused him of being a homosexual or had ever said anything about him and homosexuality?

He said "No, never."

In that case, I asked him, *"Why do you think everybody thinks you are a homosexual?*

He said "they just do."

"How do you know?"

"I just do."

"It is impossible to know what other people are thinking unless they tell you. You are just guessing and can't know".

The patient had to think about that one. He obviously had an unconscious fear that he was homosexual. This was too frightening for him to accept consciously, so he projected his fear on to everybody else making them, in his eyes, think he was homosexual. It was safer for him to think that, as he could say "They are wrong." But if he thought 'I am homosexual,' then he had no choice. I had to find out why he thought he was homosexual and reframe that, to cure him. He doesn't think he is homosexual any more.

13. 'Loss of sense of humour, inability to laugh'. Many people suffering from the effects of stress find they have no sense of humour left, and if you can get them to have a really good belly laugh it is amazing how much better they will feel. Many of my patients have said how much better they feel when I have helped them to have a good laugh, and they often say "I haven't been able to do that for ages."

Some people however use laughing as a defence, for example, when they are embarrassed, or don't quite know what to say. Others may use laughing as a defence against the threat of rising pain, again for example, when they are telling you some terrible thing that happened to them in the past. If they laugh at these times you can be fairly sure the dynamic processes of that event are still affecting them. You can get at their pain through the laugh by asking them, "What is the hurt behind that laugh"? while they are still laughing. Many of them will stop laughing and immediately begin to cry. Once again if they cry about it now it is still affecting them. Generally this laugh is different to the good old belly laugh. It's much more false.

14. 'Feeling of neglect'. Housewives feel they are neglecting their housework. Husbands and wives feel they are neglecting their partners. People feel they are neglecting their work, or their personal appearance. These are all signs of stress.

68   HOW TO BECOME THE PARENT YOU NEVER HAD

15.   'Dread of the future'. A feeling of impending doom is very common with excessive stress.
16.   'A feeling of having failed as a person or parent'. Again, these are very common feelings when stress is involved. Often the person experiencing these feelings is well respected by everyone else and the feeling in 'real terms' doesn't fit.
17.   'A feeling of having no one to confide in'. One of the most common things people say in therapy is "I have never told anyone this before", and then go on to relate some most important things in their case history. If they haven't been able to tell anyone before, the information that follows is nearly always very important and relevant to their case. This, however, can sometimes be confusing because there are patients who tell everyone they have never told anyone this before. They are just trying to get attention, and are generally third liners whose parents never listened to them.
18.   'Difficulty in concentrating'. (See 'Frank' in chapter 5.)
19.   'The inability to finish one task before rushing on to the next'. This also seems to be a very common result with highly stressed people. It is very common in second liners, for example painters who never finish a painting, often because their own feelings are in the painting. If those feelings are very negative it becomes too threatening to finish the work because they may be forced to feel those negative emotions.
20.   'An intense fear of open or enclosed spaces or of being alone'. These three feelings are often all present in the same person, and are all a result of first line traumas. (See chapter 2 on claustrophobia and agoraphobia).

There are always other symptoms, but I have covered the common ones.

As I said earlier in this chapter, the tension produced by stress very often keeps building up, so let us now look at ways of reducing stress.

Reducing Stress
  1.   Work no more than eight hours a day regularly.
  2.   Have at least one and a half days free from normal work

weekly.
 3.   Allow at least one hour for each meal before you return to work.
 4.   Eat slowly and chew well. Overweight people nearly always eat too quickly. You will see them finish before anyone else then have some more.
 5.   Cultivate the habit of listening to relaxing music.
 6.   Practise entering an altered state of hypnosis for two minutes at a time every two or three hours if you feel tense. While you are in that altered state access a relaxing scene and feel it.
 7.   Actively cultivate the habit of walking, talking and moving slowly.
 8.   Smile and respond cheerfully when meeting people.
 9.   Plan one 'away from it all' holiday each year and look forward to it.
 10.   Take regular out-of-door exercise, and deep breathe the fresh air. If playing a game like golf where you are hitting away a ball, learn to hit your tension or aggression away with it. If you don't have any game like that, then go down to the seaside or river bank and when clear to do so throw stones into the water while at the same time you are imagining you are throwing away an aggression or tension you may be feeling. Or just break old cups by throwing them away with your pent up feelings.
 11.   Examine and balance your eating patterns, and learn to enjoy the correct amount of food. Find out how much you need to maintain a healthy weight and look forward to eating that amount.
 12.   Seek advice if emotional or sexual relationships are upsetting. This is often not done because it is an area that many people are embarrassed about.
 13.   If you are unhappy at work, explore possible alternatives and when a suitable one is found, change jobs.
 14.   Cultivate a creative hobby like gardening or do-it-yourself, or painting, or acting. If, in that hobby there is some hard work to do then find a way of enjoying doing it.
 15.   Have regular massage or join a yoga or keep fit class.
 16.   Concentrate on living in the present and avoid dwelling

on the past or future for too long a period. You can only live now so make the most of each and every moment of 'now'. Don't dread some time in the future or you will programme that time to be negative. Don't dwell on some negative time from the past, otherwise you will depreciate the value of the present.

17. Work and act methodically, finish one task before starting another. As mentioned in 14 above, if some of the work is hard or boring find a way to make it enjoyable otherwise you will make it unbearable. Don't dread doing anything, for you make it harder than it really is.

18. Set attainable goals in life and when they have been achieved learn to celebrate them by feeling good about reaching them.

19. Express your feelings openly when appropriate, and if suppression is necessary, find a way to get rid of the tension that suppressing them creates, as soon as you can.

20. Do not set impossible deadlines or goals.

21. Do not rely on drugs or other people to cope with life, Become responsible for yourself.

22. Don't play the 'Blame Game'.

Do some of these things every day and learn to do them automatically so that tension is not allowed to build up in your system.

Treatment of Stress without Drugs

1. Hypnotic Techniques.

A) By relaxing techniques using visualisation of places or times when you were very relaxed.

B) By goal directed meditation with visualisation of own personal stress meter. (See below.)

C) By dissociation from stress using Spiegel's split screen technique.

D) By ego strengthening techniques.

For A, B, C and D above see the exercises at the end of this chapter.

2. Neuro-Linguistic Programming with Hypnosis.

By reframing. If a particular behaviour makes us tense, it is probable that such behaviour is not appropriate to the occasion that is causing the behaviour. It is necessary to reprogramme the way we respond to that occasion. This reprogramming is done by a process known as reframing. (See exercise below.)

3. Non-Hypnotic Techniques.

By operant conditioning. If you learn to feel good, and celebrate the good things in life. You learn by feeling good to do those things again. You don't feel tense, when you feel good.
   By Yoga.
   By meditation.

4. By Analysis.

Using analysis or hypno-analysis you can explore the dynamic factors in your unconscious mind that were responsible for the learned behaviour in the first place. (See examples in the first four chapters.) Then you may re-educate yourself to a different behaviour in a number of ways, one of which is reframing.

5. By Gestault Therapy.

By using gestault therapy it is possible, as in the case above to explore the dynamic factors in the learned behaviour and then to relearn a new behaviour more fitting to the occasion.

6. By Primal Therapy.

As in 4 and 5 above dynamic processes may be examined with primal therapy and the re-education can be done by experiencing those processes and fixing them to the event, in the past, by the reliving of the experience.

   Once again there are always other techniques, and new ones being thought of all the time. Which method should anyone use? The one which suits both the patient and therapist at the time.

EXERCISE 25. After entering hypnosis, access a peaceful relaxing scene of your own choice. Access all the feelings connected to that scene and hold on to them. Now imagine how good it would be to be wide awake, performing whatever you have to do next with those good feelings. Then just open your eyes and carry on.

EXERCISE 26.   'Goal directed meditation with visualisation of your own stress meter.' After entering hypnosis concentrate on your breathing. Become particularly aware of each breath out you take. It is relaxing to breathe out. It is like letting go of a balloon that is blown up. The sides of the balloon collapse down and the tension in the wall disappears. Breathing out is the same. When you breathe out the tension in the lung lining disappears, your lungs collapse down and the air is pushed out. Your unconscious mind is aware of the reduction in tension so you feel relaxed. You 'feel' on the nondominant side of your brain, so you feel relaxed on the nondominant side with each exhalation. You think on the dominant side of your brain so if you think of the word 'calm' and what that means as you breathe out, you both think and feel relaxed. As explained in the 'think feel' theory chapter 2 in this book it is much more efficient if you both think and feel the same thing at the same time. So if you think calm every time you breathe out, you begin to reduce tension. This is goal directed meditation.

At the same time as you are co-ordinating your breathing out with thinking "Calm" you can picture your own personal stress meter. Your stress meter can be any form of metering system that is comfortable to you, but for the sake of the description in this exercise, let us think of it like a parking meter. If you are feeling tense then you should access you meter with the penalty sign showing. Each breath out you take, while you are thinking "calm", is like putting another coin in the meter. Soon the penalty sign disappears and you feel more relaxed. If you go on co-ordinating your breathing with thinking "calm" the meter gets lower and lower, as you get more and more relaxed. Once you have lowered your tension, just like the parking meter, it doesn't immediately go up again. So if you practice this technique every few hours the penalty of feeling tense should not have to be paid, and you will become much more relaxed. Do this exercise three or four times a day for two minutes at a time.

EXERCISE 27.   Spiegel's split screen technique. In the hypnotic state, when you feel floating, access the split screen on the other side of the room. On one side see yourself tense and uptight. On the other side see yourself relaxed and calm, then tell yourself which one you want to be. Access all the feelings of the one you want to be, and bring them back from the screen leaving the 'you' you don't want on the other side of the room. Then imagine how good it will be to be doing whatever you are doing feeling like that. Open your eyes and be like that. Repeat the exercise every few hours, for two minutes at a time, until you feel well.

EXERCISE 28.   Ego strengthening. In the hypnotic state access the marathon you ran to be here. Tell yourself that you have as much right as anyone else to be here. Tell yourself that you have as much right to be as relaxed as anyone else here. Access how relaxed that can be, then open your eyes and be that relaxed. Repeat the exercise every few hours until you feel comfortable.

EXERCISE 29.   Reframing. In the hypnotic state access that part of the mind that is making you tense, in an attempt to help you cope with a situation. Ask it, when it is listening, paying attention, and willing to negotiate, to indicate that it is willing to consider change by lifting one of your index fingers. When one of your index fingers rises, thank it for its willingness to consider change and also for trying to help you cope with a situation. Respectfully remind it, however, that the way it is trying to help you, by making you tense, has become the problem. The tension is too great and, because of it, you are less able to tackle the situation.

   Then access that part of the mind which we shall call the creative part of the mind. The part of the mind which weighs up the pro's and con's of everything you do. Ask it when it is listening and wanting to help with alternatives to raise the other index finger. When your other finger rises thank it for

74 HOW TO BECOME THE PARENT YOU NEVER HAD

its willingness to help with alternative behaviours.

Now ask those two parts to get together in you unconscious mind to discuss and debate ways and means that will help you tackle the situation without making you tense. Let them be consultants for you, finding a few ways to help you cope with situations which would normally make you tense, without making you tense. Ask them, when they have found four or five ways to cope with the situations, without making you tense, to lift both your index fingers and bring them together, as a token of agreement. At this stage, because the negotiation has been going on in your unconscious mind you will not necessarily be aware of how they are going to help you. You should however find you have more options than being tense. Open your eyes and try some options. If the alternatives don't work repeat the exercise until they do.

If you want to use analysis or gestault therapy or primal therapy, it is best that you at least start with a therapist, rather than trying to do it on your own. It is very important that you choose the right therapist for you.

CHAPTER 7
Case Histories

So far I have used limited case histories to emphasise a point or illustrate a theory. In this chapter I would like to take a few case histories and follow them through from beginning to end to try to show how my theories stand up in practice. These cases are a few from the thousands I have treated over a period of twenty-five years. Naturally, over that time these theories have developed and been modified. The names used, and some of the patients' personal details have been changed slightly to protect their identity. These changes do not alter the main facts or treatments in any of the cases throughout this book.

My own personal comments throughout this chapter appear in italics.

Multiple Attempted Suicide

The first case I would like to describe is one of multiple attempted suicide, because to me it was a very important one. First of all because of the very serious nature of the case itself, but also because it taught me a great deal. The patient's name is Mary, and I received a letter from Mary's mother about her daughter on the 18th August 1977 requesting my advice regarding treatment. I am quoting her letter so that you can better appreciate all the background circumstances of this case.

Dear Mr Graham,

I received your name and address from a mutual friend who has attended a number of your courses and workshops. I was asking him about my daughter who is in desperate need of help, and he suggested that you may be able to help her. My husband and I would do anything to obtain some assistance with Mary as we are at our "wit's end".

Mary was admitted to a psychiatric ward at one of the London Hospitals in Feb. 1973 suffering from depression. She was working at the Hospital and I had been trying to contact her for about five weeks, as I had not heard from her. Eventually Mary rang me and told me where she was but I was refused access to her because she didn't wish to see me. As she was over 18 years old the hospital had not notified me and they said I could not see Mary until she agreed. Whilst on the ward Mary agreed to have Electric Shock Therapy but this produced no improvement in her mood. She also took several overdoses and cut her wrists whilst there. In May 1973 I went to visit her and they asked me to take her home, which I did, where she received anti-depressants from our own G.P. for about two weeks. Then our G.P. received a letter from the London Hospital informing him that Mary was in urgent need of psychiatric treatment so it was arranged for a psychiatrist to visit her at home.

He persuaded her to enter the local Psychiatric Hospital for one month as a voluntary patient for observation; with a promise there would be no E.C.T. (see glossary page 159) which she now both hated and dreaded. After one week she was given E.C.T. and when she objected she was told she had given permission when she signed her admittance form. During the four weeks she was there she took at least two overdoses to my knowledge, but I was not kept informed of anything. We visited Mary after one of her attempted suicides to find her in a very distressed state and on the locked ward; on her return from the Infirmary she had been put into a side room in the dark, which seemed cruel to someone who was terrified of the dark. When I asked the nurse about this I was told it was to bring her to her senses. She added that she had broken better people than Mary. At this time we were told to stop visiting Mary but I chose to ignore this request.

One evening we visited Mary after she had had a treatment earlier in the day which seemed to upset her a great deal. I begged the staff to watch her carefully as I had learned to recognise the 'danger signs'. At 11.45 p.m. I received a phone call informing me that she had jumped through a third floor window, and had been taken to casualty at the Infirmary. The outcome being multiple leg and ankle injuries and an impacted vertebrae fracture in her back. Previously the psychiatrist had said her suicide attempts were attention seeking, now he said "This girl is hell bent on killing herself. We can either put her in a padded cell for the rest of her life or wait until she succeeds in killing herself."

The Psychiatrist who was treating her wanted us to sign a form to commit her at this time, but for various reasons (including the fact that they had no facilities for nursing her) we discharged her. I felt that if I didn't take her out of there myself and take full responsibility for her safety she would never get out alive.

About a year later, when she was reasonably fit physically, we saw another Consultant Psychiatrist who treated her, again for depression, as an outpatient at another hospital for six months, after which she attended the local College and took three 'A' levels passing two of them, although she had difficulty coping at times due to recurring depression. From August 1976 to date she has again been treated as an outpatient and we seem to have reached a deadlock.

I have recently talked to the Psychiatrist and he says Mary has been given all the drugs he normally prescribes plus three, eight sessions of E.C.T. and that he considers it is rather a 'state of mind' than an illness at this time. We think there could have been some reason for Mary's illness originally which was never discovered and is causing this 'state of mind', if he is correct in his diagnosis.

Mary has, throughout her illness, had great difficulty in 'talking', in fact she seems to have withdrawn completely from everyone. She is having considerable pain from her left ankle which the Orthopaedic Consultant says cannot be treated further and that she will never be able to return to nursing or any career which entails being on her feet, all this does not help her outlook on life in the future. She has taken two overdoses in the last few months and we are obviously not satisfied that everything has been tried. We have suggested hypnosis to the Psychiatrist and he says if we can find a qualified Medical Hypnotist he has no objections, but that he is unable to put us in touch with one in Derby. She is taking no drugs at present but is working two hours a day in the Path. Lab. at the mental hospital and attending Group Therapy each day.

I hope this letter has given you an insight into Mary's difficulties and hope that you might be able to help us yourself or suggest someone in this area whom you can recommend.

I hope you will have no objections to my ringing you in a few days for your considered opinion. We would be extremely grateful for any help you can give us as we are desperate to get to the root of the trouble and find some effective treatment.

Yours faithfully,
Mrs B. M.

When Mary's mother phoned me a few days later I told her I would be willing to see Mary myself but that I practised on Tyneside and she lived in Derby. If I could help her, and I had no idea if I could until we met, she would obviously have to come for some considerable time. Her mother said if I could help her it would be worth travelling to Tyneside and she would be most grateful if I would make an appointment. I made an appointment for 3rd September 1977 and explained that I believed depression and suicide were both a result of imprinting at birth so it would be helpful if she could let me have some information about Mary's birth, together with any relevant information from her early childhood. I received the letter below by return of post, together with a letter sent to her from two of Mary's friends from her nursing days in London.

CASE HISTORIES

Letter from Mrs B. M. in reply to my request for further information.

Dear Mr Graham,

Both my husband and myself were very thrilled when we knew Mary was on the way. We had been married for two years and were living with my father-in-law at this time but he was working away from home and was only there at weekends. I was living under a great deal of tension as my father-in-law rarely spoke to me, though he was not openly hostile. However, as always he was very friendly and affectionate towards my husband. When my husband told him I was pregnant he said that we would have to find somewhere else to live as he was not taking second place to a baby. When I was about eight months pregnant, I had been away for a few days as my husband was also working away from home, I came back to find all the pipes in the house frozen and when they thawed the water came pouring through the ceiling. When my father-in-law came home there was a terrible row, and from then on my position in the house became intolerable. Whether the tension I was living under at this time would have any effect upon Mary I do not know but I think perhaps you should know about it.

Mary was born on 5th February 1954 at 12.15 a.m. in hospital. My waters had broken and I had a show at about 3 a.m. on the 2nd and I went into hospital about noon on that day. Apart from severe back-ache I had very little pain until the afternoon of the 4th, when the doctor came about 7 p.m. he said if Mary had not been born by the following morning he would do a Caesarean operation. I was left alone until I had to ring for assistance about 10.30 p.m. when the nurse told me I was about to have a baby any minute. I was taken to the delivery room and given gas and air and around midnight there was 'lots of panic' when they said the baby's heart beats were 'giving out', **(The first time Mary nearly died.)** and I was cut for a quick delivery. Perhaps I should explain that they told me Mary had not 'dropped' and the head had not become fixed as I carry my babies very high in a peculiar position and it is impossible for the head to become fixed (my son was a similar birth). I was given Mary to hold for a few minutes after which she was taken away until the following afternoon, (I was told by one of the nurses that she had cried all the time), when we were both moved to the main ward. The babies were placed at the foot of the bed in cots, but every night Mary was taken to the nursery because she started to cry about 10 p.m. and I was told she never stopped all night. **(It is my belief that she was reliving the birth, each night, that is about the time she started, and needed some comfort and got none, thus reinforcing the trauma).**

She slept all day **(A new learned defence to escape from trauma.)** and was regularly slapped on the bottom of her feet by the staff to keep her awake long enough to feed. **(Yet another trauma)** She was breast fed to three months when my milk became inadequate.

When I left the hospital I went home to live with my parents as my husband was working away and I refused to return to my father-in-law's. The same pattern continued and although Mary was in a carry-cot at the bedside the only time she slept was when I put her into bed with me, when she would sleep all night **(Womb return is safe, and before the trauma occurred.)** My husband at this time came home only at weekends.

When Mary was six months old we went to live at Newton-le-Willows where my husband was working. Mary slept in a cot by our bed and while I was holding her hand she would sleep, but as soon as I let go she would begin crying. In desperation at this time I bought her a dummy which she did not discard until she was nearly five years old. At about twelve months she developed children's eczema which she had for about two years. **(Trying to get attention Second Line.)** She appeared at this time to be a very happy child and would play for hours in the garden alone, **(It had already become safe not to feel and be away from anyone who might hurt her.)** the only trouble was at night when she would not go to bed without the light being on and never settled before 10 or 11 p.m. I did however have a lot of trouble with toilet training and had wet beds and knickers (which were frequently dirty too), this continued until after she went to school and the wet beds until she was about fourteen years, **(Unconsciously all the time trying to get attention Second Line.).** I would change her bed as many as four times during the night. **(That's when the birth trauma occurred and when she needed most attention).**

When she was two years old she had chicken pox very badly and had begun to spend a lot of time at a neighbour's house as there were no children in the vicinity for her to play with. This neighbour had no girls just two teenage boys and they all made a terrific fuss of Mary. **(At last some attention.)**

When Mary was three years old she went completely deaf and was taken into hospital to have her adenoids removed and sinuses washed. They said they had never had such a dreadful bed-wetter. **(You can imagine how much having to go into hospital at three to have your adenoids out and sinuses washed would reinforce her birth trauma. No wonder she had to try and get some attention by bed wetting.)** After this she began to have tonsilitis about every two months and we were visiting the hospital regularly. At four she started to go to Sunday School through which she became friendly with a little girl who used to come and play occasionally. For the first time we had tantrums from Mary, **(If nothing else works have tantrums. Second Line.)** mostly about sharing her toys **(She had to have something for herself that gave her joy and if that was threatened have a tantrum.)** About this time she had Whooping cough.

In 1958 my father died—I do not remember any reaction or grief on Mary's part **(She had already shut off as a result of reinforced First and Second Line trauma.)** In 1959 when Mary was almost five our son was born, she did not show much interest in the new baby but spent more time with our neighbours. **(At least they gave her the attention she craved for, and neurotically needed desperately by now.**

Third Line.) About three months later she started school and settled well. *(She might as well, she now had no chance at home with her brother being there and her at school. Third Line.)* She did not seem to be at all jealous of him. *(Already she had switched off realising her needs so what was the point?)* Her reports were good in spite of repeated absences due to tonsillitis. Her reports did say, however, that she talked too much which surprises me as Mary was always a quiet child at home. *(It is very interesting to see the report given by Mary of this time* [see later]*.)*

I remember one incident at this time. Mary had not returned from school at the ususal time and two hours later I tracked her to a child's house. The mother said Mary had told her I had said it was all right for her to go, she also told me she was very sorry to hear that we had had burlgars. This of course was not true and it was at this time I discovered Mary was telling the most fantastic lies. *(Anything for attention. If you have nothing to say say anything.)*

She then became friendly with two little girls who had come to live in the vicinity, and she played with them continuously, although she always came home very frightened because they had been telling her there were mad bulls and witches around. She became afraid to walk down the road alone, she had always been afraid of the dark but she now became terrified to go to bed and I would have to look under the bed, in the drawers and wardrobes before she would enter the bedroom. I then had to go upstairs every half hour or so to reassure her, this fear of the dark continued until she was in her teens and I believe even when she became a student nurse at the London Hospital her friends had slept with her on odd occasions because she was afraid to sleep alone she did not seem to know what she was afraid of however. *(That was too frightening* [birth] *anyhow it got some attention, being afraid.)*

When she was six she went into hospital to have her tonsils removed after which she was in bed for four weeks with a weak heart (there has been no evidence of this since then). **(Probably another birth reaction to going into hospital again. Remember at birth there was 'a panic because the baby's heart was giving out'.)** The doctor told me at this time that she was asthmatic but I did not realise this. **(Just another birth reaction.)** After this time she began suffering from inflamed ears which continued until about fifteen years of age, she was frequently at home from school with this. **(If you want attention be ill.)**

When she was seven my father-in-law died (we had become very good friends and he was extremely fond of Mary and she of him). She cried when we told her but seemed to get over it very quickly. **(She could still feel a little for others but not for herself.)** He had died very suddenly. My husband had worked away from home for quite long periods during all this time and he then took an appointment in London and the children and myself moved to Bramhall to live in my father-in-law's house. Mary was very unhappy at school at this time which reflects in her reports. **(The Blame Game, blame the school. She probably was very unhappy full stop by this time.)**

She had very few friends at this time. I should add that Mary, from the time she started school would do anything any of the children asked her and give them anything to obtain and keep their friendship, this appears to have continued as she always seems to be afraid to say no, even though she doesn't want to do something or knows she should not. **(Anything for attention and love showing a neurotic dependence had already developed.)**

We moved again, to our present address when Mary was nine. She was very happy at the school she now attended and did well again in her studies. She now had more friends and at school they said she was very responsible and reliable. She was still having ear trouble and at ten she fell and broke her arm. She passed her eleven plus and changed to the local Grammar School. At this time her bed wetting became worse again, although it improved from time to time, each time she changed classes or had new teachers it became worse. **(Mary's** *mother's claim that she was very happy, doesn't add up with her bed wetting getting worse.)* Her reports at this time always said 'Mary has real ability which she chooses not to use'. *(This is a typical remark made of Organic Brain Disfunction people. The difficult birth often results in O.B.D. and I made a note to check for O.B.D. when I saw her. This proved positive and I gave her some exercises to correct this which I will describe later.)*

When she was twelve my mother died in hospital, Mary was very upset for a short time and her periods began. Soon after this time we began to have behaviour problems, her school reports were very bad and she struck up some very undesirable friendships. On one of our visits to school several of the Staff said Mary was over-sexed, but some were more helpful and we discovered that she was being very silly asking stupid questions and being egged on by her friends but it seemed to be mostly bravado. We had a talk about it and, although we never really got to the bottom of the trouble, things seemed to improve, (the staff at school seemed to be very secretive about the trouble they were having with this Form). This is one of the periods Mary says she doesn't remember anything about. *(Third Line, memory totally blocked out.)*

Just after this time Mary had a broken finger and then she had an accident to her ankle when she had her foot trapped in a door at school. She had this stitched but it took six months to heal. She also had a suspected appendicitis and spent some time in hospital. As a result of the accident to her ankle Mary never took part in any games because it frequently became ulcerated and we were attending the hospital on several occasions for about two years. When she was fifteen she gained an 'O' level in English. At this time she with others at school became interested in the Ouija board, and really believed that she contacted spirits etc. After these sessions she became so afraid she dare not sleep alone, but she still continued to dabble with it. Mary gained seven 'O' levels when she was sixteen and entered the sixth form, but then began to do very little work for her 'A' levels. At this time I discovered she was telling lies as to her whereabouts, and was also drinking more than she told us. I also found out that she was 'going out' with a coloured boy. Later both Mary and I discovered that a friend of Mary's was expecting a baby by this same boy. Mary was genuinely upset about this and did not see the boy again although he continued to ring her for about eighteen months. Her ankle became very ulcerated at this time and she went into hospital for a skin graft. **(Second Line, skin breakdown.)** She was away from school for a term because of this, and when she returned had to drop Chemistry because she found it impossible to catch up an all her 'A' level work. She gained an 'A' level in one subject only an 'O' at 'A' level Biology. The Biology master said of Mary that because of her varying moods it was very difficult to assess her.

Mary had wanted to be a nurse for as long as we could remember and she was accepted at the London Hospital. Her father was not at all happy about her becoming a nurse but eventually gave her his blessing. A friend from school went to the London hospital at the same time and I have never known Mary to be as happy as she was for the first few months. We were so happy for her and really thought her troubles were over. Then in October I had a phone call to say Mary was being rushed to the operating theatre with an acute appendicitis. She came home on a month's sick leave and then went back on to the wards. At Christmas she rang to say she was 'off sick' with an abscess on her jaw and had had some teeth extracted.

She came home for a fortnight in January and although I knew there was 'something wrong' as she had spent most of the time in bed, **(learned in hospital immediately after birth, sleep to escape)** I never discovered what it was. She said she had swollen glands and a sore throat but I am sure there was something wrong. My husband went to see her once after she returned to London and said she seemed 'strange' and was concerned at the number of empty wine bottles she had in her room, she was also burning black candles just because she liked them, she said.

Jan. 1973. We did not hear from Mary then for about six weeks and eventually discovered (after many phone calls) that she had been in the Nurses Sick Bay for a fortnight refusing to speak to anyone and had then agreed to go into the Psychiatric ward. I heard from Mary's friend that previous to going sick they had been walking London with Mary until three and four o'clock in the morning and that she had been drinking heavily. They had also been sleeping in her room with her because she was afraid and could not sleep. They would not enlighten me any further. I am however enclosing a letter I received from Mary's friends after I discovered Mary had become interested in spiritualism through a lady she had met whilst in the Psychiatric Ward at London and asked them if they knew anything. I think I gave the relevant information on Mary's illness in my previous letter.

Yours faithfully,
Mrs B. M.

If we look at this account we can see that Mary has First, Second and Third Line traumas on top of one another, with most of them reinforced, and she has displayed behaviours learned from each, and she has also probably got Organic Brain Disfunction. One really wondered where to start, or indeed, if one should or could sort this out. Anyhow I had an appointment to meet Mary and her mother so I would see after that, what if anything, I could do. I must admit I wasn't looking forward to meeting Mary or her mother. The letter enclosed with Mary's mother's letter was from Mary's two friends in London and it appears in full below.

Dear Mrs. M.

We hope this letter will be of some use to Mary and will help clear a few matters up. Regarding the seances, Mary used to hold quite a few up until the winter holidays, sometimes with other people and often on her own as her power seemed so strong. Fran and I although literally afraid to join in, used to sit in the room when Mary wanted to hold a seance as we were worried as to what might happen and also fascinated by her ability. Usually the sequence of events was as follows: Mary would begin by removing all metal objects that she was wearing especially her cross, and would arrange the letters of the alphabet on a smooth surface, in a circle and in the centre of the circle would place a "pointer"—any object easily moved on the surface with a point to indicate which symbol the "contact" was moving towards. Often, Mary would use a bracelet, squeezed into a long oval shape. The room would be darkened or the light dimmed and those taking part (usually Kathy, who is a Quaker, and took part mainly out of curiosity and also seemed to have a strong power herself. She never wore a crucifix so never necessitated having to remove it), would sit comfortably with their index finger brushing the surface of the pointer. Mary preferred silence and also that the other people in the room removed their crosses etc. which Fran and I refused to do.

After a period of a few minutes Mary would ask if there was anybody there—usually with her eyes closed, and the principle is that if the pointer moves towards "yes" in the circle of symbols, the subsequent question must be "Are you a good spirit?" and if no answer is given then the spirit is bad and contact should be broken immediately or the evil spirit would take over the medium. If the answer was "yes" then the seance would proceed with Mary always asking the questions and then the pointer would move towards the symbols spelling out a reply.

Mary had previously, before coming to London, been in regular contact with a group from another world called "the Triffids" which may sound similar to the book, "The day of the Triffids" but this was the name of the race, and the person or being that Mary was in contact with was called "Moonie". Mary could go into great detail about their way of life, their beliefs and how they saw things—often she would have to explain her questions as certain words were not known to this being. They had in the past drawn pictures of themselves through Mary, and on one occasion asked Mary to tell us (Fran and I) to leave the room, whereupon we did and the door was locked.

Sometimes the spirits spoke only to Mary and not through the symbols, so only Mary could hear what they said, in her mind. On one occasion, Mary wanted to perform alone and although we were present, she managed to establish a strong contact and on her own seemed to sink into a trance-like state from which we could not rouse her; she was immobile and very cold. After a few minutes she spoke in a strange voice which we could not understand and we tried to rouse her, perhaps unwisely, and when she woke, she was very tired but well pleased at what had happened although had no recollection of the incident.

One evening (perhaps this is important,) Mary contacted a spirit which would not answer to the question "Are you good" but on this occasion Mary did not break contact immediately, but carried on with the seance. Also perhaps of importance, although it could be mere superstition, Mary brought a black candle just after returning to London in January, which she proceeded to burn at night, and which we threw away when cleaning her room. We both used to be sceptical of the occult until seeing Mary and we acknowledge that she does have a very real power. One factor that was always constant throughout her illness was that she would always say—"I am frightened—I don't know why I do this."

Shortly after the start of Mary's upset, Fran and I actually broached to each other that however odd it may sound we thought she could be possessed.

We hope this doesn't upset you Mrs. M. and that some good will come from this information. Give our love to Mary.

Much love,
Fran and Beth.

You can imagine with all this information regarding Mary I

was waiting with some trepidation to meet her and her mother. I must say I was very agreeably surprised when I met them. Mary's mother was a charming and most caring lady quite unlike what I had expected from the history of Mary in her letter to me. This was one of the large factors that persuaded me to take Mary on as a patient. Mary was a dumpy twenty-three year old lass about two stones overweight, totally withdrawn and uncommunicative. She avoided eye to eye contact and obviously had not been bonded with anyone. She looked down into her chest when she spoke and only mumbled a few words when spoken to. She obviously had no chance of being responsible for herself as she was being driven by an enormous amount of unresolved pain. She was completely shut off in a world of her own with excesses of fear, anger and guilt plaguing her every feeling. There was something about her that I liked, I don't know what it was, but I felt I could help her. This was the deciding factor in my taking her on. I always reserve the right to refuse a patient after we have met, as does the patient. There are a number of very necessary factors that have to be present in any psychotherapeutic relationship (see next chapter).

Mary, her mother and I went into my consulting room and talked for a while. Talking to Mary was like trying to extract an impacted wisdom tooth; every move was a struggle. I tested her for Organic Brain Disfunction and found she had no tonic neck reflex, no unilateral reflex, no crosslateral reflex and no co-ordination.

The work on O.B.D. had been done by David McGlown together with Peter Blythe in Chester. This followed some other work by Dolman and Delecato at the Institute of Human Potential in Philadelphia. David and Peter's work shows the Tonic Neck Reflex is normally present at birth, but is often absent after a difficult birth. The other reflexes develop as the child goes through the learning process of creeping, crawling and walking. These reflexes are normally present in the lower brain stem, and are used for physical co-ordination. **(Mary did complain of being clumsy, and always knocking things over.)** If these reflexes do not develop normally the person has to use higher centres of the brain, in the mid brain, to co-ordinate their physical movements, which are never as good as lower brain stem reflexes.

The main problem resulting from this, however, is not a physical one, but because the mid brain is being used for physical co-ordination it is less capable of handling behaviour at times of stress. It also prevents the full development of intellectual potential, no matter how high that may be. The patient suffering from O.B.D. will never be as good intellectually as they could be and, even worse, they will have a high tendency to breakdown at times of stress.

These factors are very largely neglected in most psychological therapies, either because of ignorance of the factors on the part of the therapist, or because the theories are not accepted by the therapist, or because preference is given to other techniques, leaving the O.B.D. as a permanent factor likely to bring about another breakdown at the next onset of stress.

I explained that, with these reflexes absent, it was like Mary was running the race of her life with an invisible pair of legs-irons round her ankles. Everyone would say she could do better but they would not be able to see the leg-irons round her ankles so they didn't know why she didn't. She would feel she was doing her best, which she was, with an invisible pair of leg-irons, which she couldn't see either, so she would feel an enormous amount of frustration. Both she, and the others, were correct in their statements but neither could see why. She was quite surprised at this statement because she said she did feel very frustrated and angry I explained that she was obviously very intelligent to have done so well in her 'O' and 'A' level's but that she would never achieve her potential while she had those reflexes absent. Fortunately it was comparatively easy to replace the absent reflexes. I showed her a set of five physical exercises for her to do for five minutes each, every day for twelve weeks which would form the absent reflexes. Before she did them I showed her how to get a carbon dioxide reflex to the brain, which would make the brain more alert and responsive, and therefore more likely to form those absent reflexes.

I felt it was imperative to pattern Mary to produce these

reflexes and also to give her something to do for herself from the very beginning of therapy, thereby involving her in her own 'cure'. This shows the patient that they are just as important as the therapist in any 'cure'; a very necessary factor in any therapeutic relationship.

I then tested her for hypnotizability which was very poor. I had expected this, as it is often the case when someone is so shut off from feeling. At this stage I decided that hypnosis was not the treatment of choice in her case, there had to be something better. I discussed Primal release therapy with Mary and her mother and told them to obtain Janov's books on Primal Therapy. By this time the hour was up so we made another appointment and I asked Mary to do the exercises I had shown her and read some of 'The Primal Scream'.

The next time she came I again tested her with the exercises I had shown her on the previous visit, to make sure she was doing them correctly. She found them very hard, as do most people, at first, when those reflexes are found not to be present.

To finish the session this time I tried some hyperventilation to see if we could penetrate any of Mary's defences. I use the term 'we', meaning Mary and I because I believe all psychotherapy is a contract between therapist and patient. It's no good one working without the other. No therapist will cure a patient by themselves. The patient has to play their part, which is equally if not more important. We got nowhere with hyperventilation on this occasion. I was still finding it almost impossible to obtain any information from Mary so I asked her to write down as much about the way she felt from as early as she could remember up to the present. Her story had to be different from her mother's. Mother's account was obviously as she saw it, but had to be flavoured with her wishes for her daughter. What is important for any patient is how the patient sees the things that are happening to them, but this is not necessarily how other people see them. There is no absolute truth but only the truth as you see it. Obviously Mary's account would be flavoured by her severe birth trauma *(making it inevitable that she would have to reject some of mother.).*

The next time Mary came she brought her own story, which I am printing out in full below to show how different it is from her mother's account. This was inevitable, and I would like to remind you that this account is written by someone being driven by massive unresolved pain.

Mary's Account of Her Life

Pre-school (under 5).

"I remember being able to hear after being completely deaf due to infected adenoids. I had both my tonsils and adenoids removed on separate occasions and I remember feeling afraid when I was being anaesthetised on one of these occasions, mainly because of the mask and its rubbery smell. I spent my fifth birthday at my grandmother's because Mum was in hospital having my brother but I can't remember him as a baby—in fact I don't think either Dad or my brother come into my memories at all. **(Father worked away, and she doesn't want to remember her brother because he was at home when she had to go to school. Third Line Trauma.)**

Over 5.

Mum threatened to leave us soon after I started school, I can't remember exactly why but I knew it was my fault **(Guilt driving her to feel this, it probably wasn't her fault at all. Third Line Trauma)**—she was wearing her coat and I was crying and clutching her coat to stop her going and I kept saying I was sorry—eventually she shut the door and took her coat off but wouldn't speak and I knew that I had to be good or else she would leave. **(She had to lie or not get found out.)** Up to this time she smacked me with her hand but then she made a birch with twigs tied together and used that. I used to try to run away and hide from her when she was going to hit me and I became very frightened of her. **(What she needed was love but got fear. Third Line Trauma.)**

About this time I had a teacher called Mr. Jones who used to rap our knuckles with a ruler and who used to make fun of me because I always started to cry before he hit me. I also remember having nightmares about this. **(Humiliation at the fear because she was already conditioned by being hit by mother. Probably it was more psychologically hurtful to be hit than the physical hurt, as this just demonstrated no love. See how well she remembers it. Third Line Trauma.)**

My next memory is of deciding to run away from home when I was about seven years old. I got home from school and said I was going out to play, instead of returning home I went to a friend's house and hid under her bed without her parents knowing—eventually my Dad came to the house and I was taken home. **(She remembers this very well showing how traumatic it must have been at the time. Many of us run away but we soon forget about it afterwards. Third Line.)**

When I was eight my grandfather died and we went to live in his house for two years. I hated the new school and built up a fantasy world. During the time we lived here, Dad was only home at the week-ends and I have a vague idea that I rather liked this arrangement.

I was ten when we moved to Derby and changed schools again. After passing the eleven plus I went to the local grammar school. When I was twelve my grandmother died and I have an idea that it was soon after this that I became disruptive at school—although it may have just coincided with adolescence. **(She became difficult, Third Line behaviour.)**

I remember very little from between the ages of ten to fifteen or sixteen. I know I was frequently ill, mainly with earache and throat infections up until the age of fourteen I think.

I was afraid of the dark all through childhood and, at some point went through a phase of being terrified of being stabbed—this was accompanied by nightmares. Until I was ten I used to insist on Mum checking the cupboards, wardrobe and under the bed for imaginary giants, witches and dragons which I believed were lurking ready to frighten me. The fear of the dark continued well into adolescence. *(The birth canal has become Giants, Witches or Dragons. Reaction to First Line Trauma.)*

There are definite blanks in my memory which old photographs, and reminiscences from Mum and Dad fail to illuminate. It is a strange sensation not to recognise yourself in old photographs and then to be told it's you. Even recounting these few memories is like talking about someone I knew only vaguely and completely unconnected to me. *(Typical of someone who has had to switch off completely and become 'Split').*

I remember feeling very much 'split' even when I was at school. I always acted the fool and got a reputation for disrupting lessons and being insolent. As punishment I was sent out of the class, given lines and was always in detention; none of which was any deterrent—the only thing which affected me was if a teacher got me on my own and tried to talk to me; that way there was no audience to play to and I usually went away and cried afterwards. I could never laugh with the others so I had to make them laugh at me instead. I did very little work at this time which made Mum and Dad angry and we were always having confrontations, especially when exams were near. I remember Dad being in tears once because I'd forgotten to bring home a Maths text book the day before an exam. I despised him for getting upset over something which seemed very trivial to me and realised that he was more concerned that I should pass exams than be happy. *(Conditional love is never any good.)* Everyone was trying to persuade me to go to University instead of doing nursing which I had wanted to do since my earliest memory. *(She can feel for others but not for herself, driving her to do nursing.)* This only made me more single-minded though I did agree to look into degree and diploma courses, and eventually settled on an integrated psychiatric and general nursing course which Dad seemed to think more prestigious than a straight S.R.N. course.

All through school Dad and Mum seemed to be only interested in what academic achievements I could make and always said that my 'bad behaviour' was due to the influence of others and the fact that they thought I was weak-willed and easily led. *(The Blame Game will get you nowhere. Most parents want what they want for their children and not what their children want. They think they know better. It never works out that way when forced upon the child.)* When 'O' levels came round I was promised money for every pass, and extra for grade one's or two's. *(The bribe is too late in life, putting too much stress on to Mary.)* I think I must have felt under a lot of pressure to do well which the doctor put down to stress and gave me tranquilisers which cured the symptoms *(teaching her not to feel again)* so he must have been right. I wasn't aware of worrying and had always believed in the easy-going image I had adopted although I knew underneath I felt unhappy and discontented. *(What she wanted was love.)* I cried with relief when I got the results but again despised my Dad for being so pleased and giving me money. *(Bought love is no good it just makes you resent the purchaser. Also teaches you to win by losing.)*

I was often off sick from school and said to be accident prone *(O.B.D. causing clumsiness.)* I also hated the discipline of the school of which the headmaster was proud—and only liked and respected a couple of the teachers. I always got on better with boys than girls and this gave me a reputation of being over-sexed, as one teacher told Mum. This resulted in her giving me a book to read, an offer to answer any questions I might have, and a testimony of 'it's not as good as it's made out to be.' *(Temptation to find out.)* I felt disillusioned with life and couldn't see any point in having anything but a hedonistic attitude which seemed to be frowned on by anyone representing authority.

I went on to do 'A' levels knowing that I didn't need to pass them and still being rather disruptive. I made many resolutions to work hard but was easily distracted, couldn't concentrate very well and didn't believe I was particularly clever anyway. *(By this time she was conditioned, she only did it for them. She now had to think she wasn't a very nice, or clever person; a further part of the conditioning.)*

I first admitted to myself that I wasn't very happy when I became friendly with John who was a year older than me—I was now 17. He made me talk seriously and wanted to know me, which I found frightening because I couldn't find anything inside. It was at this time that I made a second suicide attempt by trying to cut my wrist. I only made a small cut because I couldn't find the courage to do it properly. **(This attempt was a call for help.)** John told me he loved me, which scared me and partly because of this and also because my parents liked him (especially Mum) I finished with him. **(That which you have always wanted but have never had becomes too painful to have.)** For some time I had preferred their disapproval to approval. **(Rationalisation of if I can't get love I'll have hate. At least that's attention.)**

After this I got friendly with Valerie and used to go out drinking with her on Saturday lunchtimes. To finance these trips I used to steal money from Dad without any qualms. It was through Val that I met Bevin who was West Indian and who had a pregnant girlfriend who I knew vaguely at school where she was in the year below me. I knew there could be no deep involvement and got pleasure from knowing Mum and Dad would be shocked if they found out. Bevin asked me to go to bed with him—I refused and eventually told him I was a virgin. I had been uptight about this for some time and eventually decided to satisfy my curiosity. Bevin was ideal for this because he was almost a stranger to me and could make no emotional demands. (It was safe because I wouldn't have to 'feel'.) The whole thing was pretty disastrous because he kept losing his erection but eventually I was deflowered. I had been lying to Mum and Dad in order to meet him, though I think I had told Mum I was going out with someone. Then Bevin's girlfriend rang Mum and told her I was seeing the father of her child and I had to tell them both that I hadn't known about this. I had to finish the relationship and I was not allowed to go out for quite a while.

The next year is a bit hazy but includes Mum finding out that Valerie had to go to the V.D. clinic and putting pressure on me to break the friendship. I was drinking heavily whenever the opportunity arose and became fascinated by drugs which I tried, unsuccessfully, to obtain. I did very little school work, became friendly with Gill and started dabbling in the occult and making myself frightened by it. I only passed one 'A' level which didn't please Dad but I was surprised that I had even done that because I had done virtually no work for the exams.

Then I went to London and felt a short-lived sense of freedom when my parents left. My memory of this time is very patchy and I can't get things in chronological order. G. who had been at school with me was one of the 16 who started this new course at the same time as me. We weren't particularly friendly at school but were thrown together by this common factor in London.

I resented G for being homesick and she would often say she had a headache or was too tired when we had arranged to go out. I still kept the extrovert and carefree front and I can't remember just when this began to slip. I know it was shortly after I had my appendix out.

I can only remember the signs that something was wrong and feeling that everything was falling in pieces around me. These signs were—heavy drinking and never wanting to be sober, **(It was safer to be drunk, the pain was now too near the surface and she couldn't hold it back without something.)** a constant fear of hallucinating (which was put down to the recommencement of an interest in the occult), inability to concentrate and being unable to organise things like laundry, meals and work which should have been done.

I was taking the Pill at this time and I was sleeping with two or three male nurses who I had been friendly with. I think this was the only way I could feel near to anyone and the fears would go for a while. It never occurred to me that I was ill but someone—perhaps Bill a medical student who I talked to—persuaded me to see one of my tutors who said I should see the doctor in the sick bay.

She said I was suffering from depression and admitted me to the sick bay where I saw a psychiatrist. He prescribed M.A.O.I.'s **(Anti depressants)** and a week or so later I cut my wrists with a glass I had broken. I think this was just after my nineteenth birthday and was probably only done to express how helpless and scared and desperate I felt. After this they said I would have to be admitted to a psychiatric ward and gave me a choice of three hospitals. I chose the unit which was in the main hospital.

I now rang home and said I had depression but that I didn't want them to come. After I was admitted I refused to eat for a while, cut my wrists on two occasions, had E.C.T., **(Electric Shock Therapy)** got drunk nearly every night, took barbiturates and other downers, took several overdoses of aspirin and paracetamol, had sex with anyone I could, went out with a junkie, was still scared of hallucinating, tried to drown myself and suffocate myself and generally got into a mess. They tried keeping me confined to the ward but I took a bottle of paracetamol out of Mum's bag when she came once and another time I conned Dad into fetching a bottle of aspirin from the chemist—both I took as an overdose. By this time my stomach kept haemorrhaging from the aspirin and my veins were in a mess from the drips and blood tests I'd had to have.

Eventually, after discharge and readmission, the doctor persuaded me to go home. Then I saw another psychiatrist who admitted me to hospital. He originally said I was schizophrenic and later that I was psychotically depressed. Here I had two courses of E.C.T., insulin therapy and numerous different anti-depressants and tranquilisers. I wouldn't eat or talk much. I was more or less tricked into signing the consent form for E.C.T. and prevented them doing the first few by telling them I had eaten. I saved up my tablets twice, took them as overdoses and so was put on the locked ward for a few weeks. After this I took a bottle of paracetamol which I took from Mum's handbag again.

While I was in that hospital I felt nothing except when I

was recovering from the anaesthetic after E.C.T. when I would cry. Then I had abreaction with sodium amytal followed by injections and largactyl. I think it must have been around midnight *(about the same time of day as she was born)* when I jumped out of the window. For a while when I was on the ground, I thought I was dead or about to die. *(Remember she had just jumped out of a third floor window. She had gone to the toilet because the ward windows didn't open, but the toilet one did. This was no cry for help, this time she really meant it.)* Then I realised that was not the case. I tried to get up and then felt the pain in my back and legs. I remember feeling frustrated and angry and wanted to just get up and go inside so that no-one would know. Then I got frightened and wasn't sure again whether I was alive or not and then I screamed and started crying. Mum and Dad were at the hospital when they wheeled me in and I was crying and kept saying "I'm sorry."

Most of the time in the infirmary is a blank but at the beginning I remember that I shouted for pethidine *(a very strong pain killer)* everytime I woke because I didn't want to be conscious. *(A feeling she relived after a rebirth in therapy with me.)* I also remember the sister telling me I had to eat and then being sick after a couple of mouthfuls of minced chicken. From then onwards I couldn't keep anything down. *(She had now become anorexic.)*

I was then transferred back to the psychiatric hospital. It was at this time Mum and Dad were told that the psychiatrist wanted to put me on section 25 *(commit her to a mental hospital)* for an initial six months to do a long term abreaction. The sister also expressed the opinion that I would be dead in a few months if I didn't start eating and that I should go somewhere else to convalesce before any more psychiatric treatment. So my parents discharged me. *(She was very anorexic at this stage.)*

I was flat on my back at home for a few months and being fed on baby food which I eventually started to keep down. It took a long time of physiotherapy before I could walk and only then discovered I'd broken my back, ankles, toes and one leg. At the start I kept fainting with the pain and all the way through I felt it was pointless because I didn't want to live anyway.

The next psychiatrist I saw said I was to go to a day unit but didn't want to risk admission as an in-patient due to the case history. I couldn't talk to him either but had a sort of spiel which I could reel off about symptoms. A few days before I saw him I took an overdose of chlorpromazine and tofranil which were in the cupboard—this wasn't discovered and I just felt awful the following day.

At the day unit there was group therapy again. I couldn't talk about myself. The psychiatrist went through all the anti-depressants again including various combinations. There was a six-month limit here and I was discharged after this time.

The condition for the discharge was that I get a job or something. I decided to retake 'A' levels and then do psychology at university. The first couple of months at college were bad because I had started one and a half terms late and was three or four years older than most of the others in my group. I didn't want to talk to anyone and I spent most of the days working. After Christmas I met Tom who was two or three years younger than me, though I didn't know that for a while. I knew a few people by this time but was getting depressed and suicidal again. I became very dependant on Tom and lived only through him. Life at home got steadily worse as I went out more and more and I did hardly any work. After about nine months I started to drink a lot and using pain killers to deaden myself. Tom had changed a lot and become possessive and disapproved of my drinking habits and by now I was using any medicines that I could buy that would dope me—sometimes I would drink a bottle of cough medicine with a bottle of wine in an afternoon. I'd started drinking spirits too. Then I started having sex with other people as well as Tom.

During this time the last psychiatrist asked me to go back to the day unit, I refused and so he gave me more pills. After nearly two years Tom and I split up (I was now 22) Dad disliked him from the start and both Mum and Dad thought I should be working instead of going out. I think I was probably on the road to alcoholism by now. I had been offered two places to do psychology but I knew I couldn't take another failure. Somehow I managed to pass two 'A' levels.

Relations with my parents were non-existent after rows about going on holiday with Tom and his family, going away at Christmas, staying out all night coming in drunk and not working. I'd had to steal money again to finance everything and I think they suspected my brother. They also disapproved because I'd gone to the 'Rock Festival' (where I had taken the drug L.S.D.).

I took another overdose when Tom and I split up and got caught by Mum who gave me salt water. I agreed to return to the day unit. For the last six months I'd been wetting the bed on and off which I found very distressing and embarrassing. **(A return to Second Line behaviour.)**

I went back to the day unit where I had E.C.T. again, more drugs also some one-to-one talks with the staff nurse which weren't very successful. I was still going once a week to a Folk Club and usually getting paralytic. Just before Christmas I came home from there and took an overdose of distalgesic **(another pain killer)** which I don't understand why or how was discovered but I spent a couple of days in hospital. Dad always took me to the Folk Club and collected me in the car and it was easier not to argue. After a while I stopped going.

After I had been at the day unit for six months the psychiatrist said I was to work in the Path lab. every morning, to prepare me for getting a job on discharge. I got on quite well with the woman who ran the lab. and eventually I was taking blood and doing everything she did. I took a needle and syringe and tried to inject air into my vein once, but I couldn't get into the vein.

It was then I discovered I had hypoglycaemia **(low blood sugar)** and I went into hospital for a week or so of tests which showed that my blood sugar level stays constantly low—they said the only cure would have been to remove some pancreatic tissue but that was much too dangerous. It was immediately after this that I had an operation to straighten my toes. I got them to prescribe pethidine **(Strong Pain Killer)** after the operation. Afterwards the doctor gave me the D.F.118. **(Another Pain Killer.)** All these drugs make me feel numb and seem to reduce the despair and death-wish and this makes the days easier to get through.

Most of this account is superficial and there are many more things too sketchy or too difficult to write about. I don't think I've included every suicide attempt either.

I'm still almost obsessed with self-destruction and fantasise about how to kill myself or going somewhere isolated and just living until I die. Sometimes I wish Mum and Dad were dead and at times I feel I could kill them myself. I think I feel ashamed for hurting them such a lot.

When I was a child Mum wouldn't allow any display of anger or fear or any emotion. She frequently used to say that children should be seen and not heard and we weren't allowed to criticise her or be impolite in any way. I have memories of being smacked and not knowing why and I think I was afraid of Mum. I was always telling lies—I think mainly to try to avoid a spanking. They always tried to stop 'bad behaviour' with threats or rejection. **(Third Line Trauma.)**

Now it's silence and tight lips to prevent me doing something which is disapproved of. No-one ever talks straight—its all manipulations and hiding feelings and insinuations. Maybe I'm the same. I also have the impression that I wasn't allowed to make a mistake without a warning from Mum or Dad. When I was little it was 'be careful you'll fall' and later 'you'll be sorry if you don't work now and get 'O' levels'. Even now they only point out the disadvantages and bad points of something, never acknowledging the advantages".

For someone who couldn't talk about herself at all, she had just done a pretty good job of writing about it. The trouble was where does one start with a case like this. She was bound to be anchored to failure now by all the unsuccessful previous attempts at therapy. The fantastic quality and clarity of how she saw it, in her account, made me feel I had to come up with something special, but what could one come up with now? I asked her about her seances with her friends while she was in London, again she had difficulty in talking about them. I went through her account with her and she was unable to add anything of value. I checked her O.B.D. exercises with her. She was still having difficulty with them, showing how much these movements were foreign to her. She told me she was very clumsy and was always knocking things over. I tried some more 'Hyperventilation' with her, explaining to her, that this form of therapy oxygenated the brain and broke down some of the 'Primal Gates' against pain so it might loosen up her defences and allow her to 'get into some feeling, so that we could resolve it. I tried her in both 'Reichian, and Alexander Lowen', positions while hyperventilating but still couldn't get her to feel anything. I then decided I would have to resort to more 'difficult to resist' symbols with Mary, because if we were going to be successful with any treatment I would have to teach her to 'feel'. I obtained a guarantee from both Mary and her mother that if Mary committed suicide successfully I would not be blamed as she had already tried with many of her other therapists. This was freely given, together with a promise that if Mary was to try she would first talk to me, on the phone, or by whatever means she could. I decided that the most pressing thing to treat was her suicide attempts, because, if she succeeded in this, there wasn't much point in treating any other of her traumas. In my opinion suicide is always a behaviour learned at birth so I decided to try a rebirth next time. Depression is also a learned birth behaviour so we could attempt to 'kill two birds with one stone' if you will forgive the expression. I told Mary we would try this when I saw her the following week.

The next time I saw Mary she said she had written an explanation of her experiences with the 'ouija board'. See below.

"I have decided to write this account of my experiences of spiritualism and the 'ouija board' to clear up certain discrepances in versions. I feel that these incidents have got rather out of proportion and have been given too much emphasis and importance. This is probably due to the fact that, at one time, my mother was convinced that my depression was a direct result of these things. I think this was partly because of her religious beliefs and also because there was a great deal of publicity concerning the film 'The Exorcist' and the effects that occultism was supposed to have on mental health. I am sure that, at one point, she was seriously considering exorcism even though we very rarely discussed the subject, or my experiences. That is not to say she had no grounds for her belief and it is these I wish to clarify.

The whole thing started when my friend's boyfriend was 'on leave' from the Navy and persuaded the two of us to take part in an seance with him. Apparently this was a regular pastime on board his ship and he went into considerable details about their experiences and said they were regularly in contact with intelligent plants, on a planet, who called themselves Triffids. At this time I had never heard of the book of the same name. We had a seance during which these 'plants' were introduced; hence the rather dramatic statement that 'I thought I was in touch with another planet'. I was certainly very emotionally involved, although not entirely convinced, which resulted in an almost obsessional search for proof by myself and my friend. I think it was probably this doubt which resulted in me becoming terrified of being alone or in darkness **(Not so, she was afraid before this of being in the dark, but a good rationalisation, because the truth, 'birth trauma' was too painful to feel.)** for perhaps two months, at that time. **(The 'unknown' was probably what triggered off the fear which was the same at birth.)** Sometimes I had to wake Mum and ask her to sleep with me, because I felt threatened by this invisible and incomprehensible 'force'. The fear of the dark was also reminiscent of childhood. **(You bet it was!)**

I recovered from these anxieties quite some time before starting nursing in London. *(Managed to push them out of consciousness.)* After about four months in London I started with depression and began desperately searching for something to believe in. *(She now needed another defence.)* I had more or less rejected Christianity when I was around 16. I wanted to believe in the 'occult' and consequently began having seances again. Once again I became afraid of the dark and solitude and had to rely on friends to support me after becoming unable to cope with it. *(It had come back into consciousness for the same trigger.)* Then the incident, to which the letter from my friends referred, occurred. This is the first time I have confessed to the truth behind this. *(She is beginning to trust me so I must be getting somewhere.)*

I wanted to convince my friends that the spirit world existed because—I don't really know why—I just wanted them to be 'with me' *(That's right, the new chosen defence. If someone is with me I can't feel being born because I experienced that as if I was all alone.)* close to me. I tried to do this by pretending to go into a trance and speaking in 'tongues' and delivering 'spirit messages'. I suppose I was successful in a way because they took it seriously but regarded it as an evil and tried to stop me going any further with it. Again I am not trying to minimise the effect the whole lot had on me—I was terrified for quite some time after this, even when admitted to the psychiatric ward. *(When you don't 'feel' you are only half conscious so it is difficult to tell what is the truth and what isn't, even when you start the lie. You have to keep it up or get found out, and she had learned not to get found out a long time before, so she had to begin to believe it herself.)*

Perhaps all these things do add up to seeking attention *(They certainly do, but that had become your defence so you had to have somebody there otherwise you were alone and would begin to feel the First Line Trauma.)* but the incident above was the only piece of deliberate deception I undertook. *(Guilt now, but really she had no choice as her*

First Line Trauma was now driving her to this defence.)

I also kept the fact that I was involved in spiritualism very much to myself, and the few people who I wanted to be with me, which has probably led to a certain amount of supposition on the part of my mother. ***(If you don't understand something, invent it, but it is nearly always magnified out of all proportion. See text on children being sent away from arguing parents.)***

The only times I spoke of it was when the terror became unbearable when I would usually just say "I am afraid of the spirits, will you sleep with me?"

(She had to believe it or get found out, anyhow it gives her an unconscious reason for having her defence of having somebody there.)

At least this account gives the other side of the story, although the idea that I may have believed that I was communicating with the dead and plants seems silly to me now, and perhaps I consequently underplay it. ***(No, you are just becoming more truthful with yourself. The first sign that you will get better.)***".

After going through all this I didn't think I had time to do a rebirth so we did some more loosening up exercises. Perhaps Mary was unconsciously trying to delay the rebirth because she was still too afraid.

I was having some difficulty in getting Mary to talk during the sessions so I had asked her to keep a diary of how she felt, and any other relevant details. As you have seen, her written accounts were excellent. The next time she came I decided to try a rebirth with her. I placed a mattress on the floor and asked her to lie on top of it. She then did some hyperventilation to oxygenate her brain for a short time, and then I placed another mattress on top of her. This second mattress I held down on top of her and I asked her to try to get out. I managed to prevent her getting out for some time and she often gave up trying. Each time she gave up I persuaded her to try again. In the end after she was fairly exhausted, I let her get out, and then held her as you would a baby. As Mary hadn't been bonded, I would look at her and ask her to look into my eyes. She found this almost impossible to do, saying that she could only see emptiness in my eyes, and that it was very hurtful to her. When I was looking into her eyes I was thinking as hard as I could that I loved her and wanted her to be here, (born) as I had often done with my own children; not because my own children hadn't been bonded, but because I loved them. Her feeling, therefore, that she could only see emptiness that hurt her must have been a reflection of what she felt inside herself. It is essential after doing any regressive action with symbols that you 'bottom' the patient afterwards. This means give them something good to go away with and give them time in a safe atmosphere to come back to the present time no matter how much regression they manage to achieve with the symbolic conditions. Hence the need to hold them lovingly, as you would your own children.

She didn't say much afterwards but looked fairly shattered. It was also very different from anything she had ever experienced with any other of her psychiatric therapies. This point was important, as it would be too easy for her to think here we go again, 'they aren't going to make any difference by doing that'. As she had never experienced anything like this she was unable to reject it out of hand.

The next time she came she said she had had a dream. This is what she had written down.

There was a loud, whistling noise accompanied by a feeling of pressure on the side of my head. There was a man's voice saying "I'm not sure" and an ambulance siren every few minutes. I felt increasing discomfort and felt that I was trying to turn over but kept being pushed back again. There was a feeling of fear until a light came which grew stronger and I was struggling to do something'. She had also written Tuesday: Bit more talkative today. Felt generally tense and lethargic still. My concentration is pretty bad and also my memory.

Wednesday: Headache again but a little better on the whole, i.e. not so depressed. It takes very little to make me 'shut off' though. I'm tired all the time and seem to have hardly any energy.

Thursday: Depressed again today and irritable. Cried for a very short time this afternoon. The rest of the week was a repeat of Thursday". She had obviously 'shut off' again. The next time she came I rebirthed her again in the same way and tried again to form a bond but once again she was unable to accept the bond.

Her report of the week "—feeling very bewildered, empty and anonymous. Headache bad. Glad to go to bed and sleep. Feel tearful but can't cry.—Quite deeply depressed, irritable and want to be on my own.—Cutting myself off from everyone and just want to sleep.—Hurting everywhere and finding it difficult to eat. Was a bit less depressed after a few days". The day before her therapy: "—I've had a headache all day but a little less depressed. Felt alienated from everybody somehow."

I rebirthed her again, and again was unsuccessful at bonding. Her report.

I seemed to ache all over especially shoulders, neck and stomach. Headache came on on the way home. I feel emotionally drained and physically exhausted. I'm getting panicky about Christmas—I don't know what I hate about it—and kept remembering that last year, the night before Christmas Eve, I took an overdose. I know it won't happen again but it keeps coming up too often for comfort. **(She is now beginning to see she doesn't have to kill herself.)** Quite depressed and a bit sensitive. People seem to be getting at me and criticising me. I have never liked people getting annoyed with me. Have been withdrawn but less anxious, but from time to time quite depressed".

I repeated the previous week's treatment with the same failure to establish a bond.

"After treatment felt completely exhausted and numb and I keep drifting off into a world of my own. The next day I woke up shivering and sweating at the same time, my guts are in a knot and my stomach is turning over. I think it's fear. I have cried two or three times—just a few tears. Afterwards I felt depressed but not as bad as last week and I think a little less afraid. I have to keep fighting the depression. Stomach still tense and a little light-headed".

Repeat therapy.

"Shattered as usual. Tense but not anxious, just numb. Felt a bit suicidal on Christmas Eve but didn't really think how I should do it.—Thank goodness Christmas is over. I smiled a few times tonight and attempted to laugh as well. Quite a bit better next day. I was quite cheerful tonight and managed to laugh a bit with everyone else. It's a pity to spoil it but I feel quite depressed now I'm in bed. Feel not too good again today and have had to collect some sleeping pills and painkillers just to deaden things. I don't want to do anything stupid when there seems a good chance of getting well, which there's never been before.—I gave up last night and took a sleeping pill. I've felt as if I went through a birth again and short of screaming it was the only way out as I feel so alone and afraid at night, even if someone is in the room. I felt much better the next day though".

"I felt depressed during today's session and felt like I was giving up. The pain in my chest was bad. (Mum says my heart was very weak so perhaps there actually was pain there.) I just didn't want to 'come out'. I've still got that pain in my back and in my shoulders now.— Depressed in the morning and afternoon but am a lot better tonight. I keep on losing track of time, I suddenly notice I have been totally unaware of the previous ten minutes or so. Still got the pains in my shoulders".

We went on in this vein, rebirthing her over and over again and getting a little more information as we went on. In one of her sessions she said it was as if she was being rubbed all over with sandpaper while she experienced her birth. Her report after read 'It felt as though I was being pushed through a tube of coarse sandpaper: dry and gritty with a dragging or pulling sensation all over on my skin'. She had had a dry birth as her mother's waters had broken three days before (see mother's account of birth at the beginning of this chapter). Her shoulders were frequently painful during and after her rebirth which would indicate her depression started when she had got her head through the pelvic arch and when her shoulders were stuck and unable to get through. After one session, she said all the way home in the train, she could feel as if her body belonged to her, a feeling she could not remember ever having before that session. After about one hour of feeling that her body belonged to her, she said, she got frightened and stopped feeling like that, and went back to not feeling. I considered this was a breakthrough, because if we were to get anywhere we had to get her to start to feel again permanently.

Round about this time Bill Swartley, the president of the International Primal Association, was paying me a short visit, and he had a session with Mary. He felt she had 'given up' at some point in her birth and had probably become unconscious. Following this she had not wanted to live any more. He told me privately afterwards that he thought I had taken on an impossible case, but if I could get a result in her case I should be able to help anyone. I must admit there were times when I felt we were getting nowhere. Mary's mother had told me that Mary's biggest fear was that I would get sick of treating her and stop therapy. If that happened Mary said she was lost for ever.

It was about this time that, following rebirthing, Mary would spontaneously produce bruising in various parts of her body, but especially round her eyes and on her face. Many of those bruises and swellings were similar to those she had after her birth. On many occasions, about two days after her session, she would say her face was sore around the eyes and her brow bones felt bruised and swollen. They were like that at the time of her birth. In one of her reports she says, "I have been reading the section on drugs and their effect on consciousness in Janov's PRIMAL MAN, and have realised why I rely so heavily on my analgesics, which are codeine mostly. Janov says that codeine acts on first line pains, together with barbiturates—which I also found effective. It took quite an effort to admit to myself that I am often taking analgesics when my physical pain is not really too bad, and even taking double doses when my defences are thin; i.e. if I feel tense or anxious and when particularly depressed. I realise how dependant on them I have become and how difficult it would be to get through the day without them".

Again on many of her sessions she experienced pain, anxiety, stomach tension, almost unbearable back and shoulder pain accompanied by a feeling of 'I can't stand this' and 'I'm going to die' and 'I want to die to escape this!'

If you remember her mother's account of the birth she had been given gas and air so I tried some relative analgesia (gas and air) with Mary, and on each occasion she experienced very strong feelings of 'I want to die to escape this hell". After each of her sessions while I was holding her I would tell her the birth was over and she need not feel like that any more. I told her that her suicide feelings were left over feelings from birth and as that was now over she could stop feeling them. I also explained that when she stopped feeling at birth she probably saved her life as the pain had been so great, but as it was over now, it was much safer to feel. Gradually and very slowly she began to feel more and more.

Langa in his book Relative Analgesia in Dental Practice, says one of the disadvantages of using Relative Analgesia is that sometimes patients experiencing R.A. will spontaneously start to cry for no reason. I believe R.A. has the ability to break down the Primal Gates to pain and those patients who spontaneously cry are experiencing some pain from a past event. General anaesthetic can also have this effect. This is why I found R.A. useful in Mary's case.

After another of her sessions she experienced an intense hostility, almost hate, towards her mother. During that time she wanted to hurt her mother physically or mentally and felt like literally tearing her into pieces. She felt very guilty about this, so I explained that it was a very natural reaction when you think that someone has just tried to wipe you out. As her mother actually had not tried to wipe her out and wanted her safe and well, and as it was nobody's fault that the birth was difficult, she could stop trying to hurt her mother. For a number of times after this she felt this hostility towards her mum which she said was so unfair and unreasonable. In the end however this hostility began to subside. This enabled Mary to see that on many occasions it had been her fault, and not her mother's, in many of the arguments they had had all her life.

In one of her reports she described depression as though it will never end whereas 'good days' always feel fragile and almost on the brink of depression, very thin and totally unreal. I explained that in birth if you chose to stop feeling as a defence to the pain, and if you have not got any further in the birth when you start to feel again, you become afraid to feel and wish that you will never feel again; hence the feeling that depression will never end, and it is unsafe to feel. **(Learned behaviour.)**

Her report goes on to say "I have been thinking about being 'ducked' in the swimming pool in London and am sometimes convinced that it started this depression in some way—(perhaps triggering of birth pains). Sometimes, especially in bed in the dark, I remember it vividly: three male nurses who I knew well did it and held my arms and head while I was under water. I remember thinking I was going to die, struggling, feeling helpless because I couldn't move much and then deciding to relax and just let it happen. I was terrified for a while but that went and it felt as though they were squashing my head. When they let me up I was choking and crying and I felt very angry towards them. I explained this was over and she could 'feel' again as it was safe to do so. **(This had probably been a reinforcement of the original birth trauma.)** She went on to say in one of her reports that some of her feelings are very hard to think of as just memories from birth, in fact if she had not experienced them on rebirthing she would have found it impossible to do so.

On one occasion her brother was fooling about and put his hands round her neck and squeezed gently. She immediately felt as though she was suffocating, got frightened and then had a headache and felt pains in her jaw and round her eyes and shoulders. Afterwards she felt very angry with him and wanted to hurt and frighten him in return. Once again this made her very aware of how, on many occasions, she had over-reacted in her life, causing herself more pain as a direct result of that over-reaction. For some time after this episode, she felt her brother hated her and she wanted to hurt him back, but she couldn't so it just built up inside her and made her more irritable.

She states in another report, following a rebirth, that she felt sick in her stomach, her chest felt tight and sort of crushed, and during the night it felt bruised, together with her face and shoulders. Several times that night she had the feeling that her heart was going to stop and that she was unable to breathe. Certain noises triggered that feeling off; like fast echoing footsteps—which, in retrospect reminded her of the tape of birth sounds which I sometimes played during her rebirth. Another time she felt it was when a train went into a tunnel or passed another train at speed. She was now realising that there were many anchor situations where her birth feelings were being triggered off. Another time she reported "After therapy I usually feel as though something has opened in my brain which then slowly closes again". I would have to find a way of keeping her brain 'open' or 'feeling' if we were going to make a permanent change with Mary.

Another time after a rebirth she found when she got home she hated everybody, and despised them for not hating her, or at least for showing her nothing but kindness and patience. She had always felt that if they didn't care or weren't alive she could kill herself more easily whenever she wanted to. This helped her to see why she resented people who had tried to talk to her and help her, and why she had rejected all their efforts at helping her. As a result of this she didn't like herself very much. I had to help her to see that it was through the faulty perception she had at birth that she was having to react like that, and it was no use blaming herself. She would have to learn to like herself.

It was about at this time, unfortunately not recognised by

me, that she got stuck in a primal rut. She felt very bad after one of our sessions, very suicidal, in a great deal of pain and very depressed. We continued with the rebirthing, thinking she would feel what it was all about but she just got worse. I now recognise that she was continuing to feel her birth more and more, over and over again when she probably had felt it enough, and rebirthing her at that stage just anchored it more, and was making her feel worse. She was probably feeling the pain of the rebirth rather than that of her birth. At this time she lost a lot of weight and had become anorexic. This went on for about three months and in the end out of desperation I decided to try something else. This was a lesson I learned the hard way, that is, if something doesn't work: do something else. As a therapist you have always got options, or you should have, so if one thing doesn't work, do something else. The only thing that comforted me during this time was that Mary never lost hope entirely, and never tried to end it all. We must have made some progress because in the past she would have tried many times to commit suicide.

By this time I had bonded with Mary and she could look into my eyes, and she was communicating a little more verbally. I decided to try some hypnosis again. Much to my surprise her hypnotic capacity had increased quite considerably. I talked to her about the Marathon, and the Journey and the Purpose of Life, telling her that if she didn't make it this time she would just have to do it all over again. This didn't seem to have much effect consciously and she used to say that is a load of rubbish, but as I was doing this in a hypnotic state her unconscious mind, or something that I didn't recognise, made her change direction and come out of the primal rut into which she seemed to have got stuck.

She began to eat again and feel less suicidal. It was now about a year and a half since I had started working with Mary. As she began to 'feel' a little more I worked with her to see if we could help her child, (The birthing child, and young child and adolescent girl) to grow up. We did this by reframing her behaviour, and in all the ways described earlier in this book. Slowly she became more independent and adult and then realised that she was now nearly twenty-five years old with no real means of supporting herself. I arranged for her to see David McGlown in Chester as another part of his work was to do educational assessments, as well as his work with O.B.D. Both Mary and I now felt it was imperative that she begin some sort of training course to gain her independence, but she didn't know what on earth to do.

David did three education assessment tests with her and provided a report with a list in order of preference of the sort of courses she should be able to cope with. He agreed with me that Mary was very intelligent and should be able to do well.

Mary wrote away to enquire about a variety of courses, and eventually went to university to study drama. Her mother was apprehensive as Mary had tried so many things in the past, only to fail and get depressed. I reassured her things would be different this time, as did Mary; and I arranged to see Mary during her half term and end of term holidays. I also made her some tapes on becoming your own parent, as in the text of this book, which she would play to herself while at college.

She completed her course with flying colours and only came up to see me during her holidays. Unfortunately at the end of her course she could not get any work and the university offered her a postgraduate course but she decided to do something entirely different. When she completed this new training she got a job and has been fully employed ever since.

When I decided to write this book I contacted both Mary and her mother to seek their permission to include her in my case histories. A letter from Mary's mother, and one from Mary herself, give details of the current situation and both letters appear in full below.

Mary's mother's letter dated September 1985.

Dear Mr. Graham,

Mary has now been in full time employment for nearly two years, thoroughly enjoying her job and admits to amazing even herself as to just what she is capable of. She is now completely independent, living a long way from home and can cope with anything.

Her weight is stable, and she eats normally, plays squash, table tennis and skittles which is surprising when you consider that she had so little co-ordination prior to her illness, she couldn't even catch a ball. In fact she works very hard and plays hard. She now has lots of confidence, makes her own decisions, speaks her mind and is able to communicate with anyone. Her friends also say they can talk to her as she is a really understanding person.

Friends of the family who have known her most of her life don't recognise her as the same person and seeing photographs of her during her illness say she looks like a zombie, now she is really alive and looks like the intelligent person she is.

The skin graft she had before her illness and which was so obvious when you were treating her has almost faded and she now takes no tablets at all.

I would not like to live through those years again, but looking back now, both Mary and I say it was worth it. She really is a different person and capable of so much more than she had ever been in her life. We shall always be grateful to you for all you have done for Mary and particularly for caring when we so desperately needed someone to care. For the first time we were treated as people and not just another case.

Thank you,
Yours,
Mrs. B. M.

Mary's letter dated Sunday 6th Oct. 1985.

Dear Geoff,

Writing this letter is not the easiest task I've ever had, but here goes.

Before the primal therapy I don't think I ever reacted to the real current situations—I would either switch off altogether or else trigger off feelings totally irrelevant to what was really happening. I felt very negative about everything, never thinking about the future and incapable of proper relationships—not very surprising because I never felt I actually knew myself and wouldn't let anyone else.

I now know myself very well and react to things in a real way—I'm now aware of how I feel and can accept and cope with my feelings. I'm working as a computer programmer, a job with plenty of pressure and stress—I now know when I'm under stress and cope with it in a positive way:—by removing the source if I can, a hard game of squash or talking to someone about the problem. Previously I would have thought 'I can't cope with this' and switched off completely and probably thought about killing myself.

I have a very good relationship with my boyfriend who I've known for two years; I feel I can be totally honest and open with him because it is a real relationship—I am no longer afraid of rejections or losing security. We regularly have friends saying how envious they are and asking for advice! I could never have had a relationship like this before because I was always so busy trying to satisfy unreal needs that I could never trust anyone or repect their needs and give as well as take.

There are so many differences between now and then because it's only in the last five or six years that I've experienced emotions relating to 'now' and appropriate to 'now'. I now not only know myself but respect and love myself; there may be things that I don't like too much but I can accept that they are a part of me and best of all I feel 'real'.

>	Thank you and
>	lots of love,
>	from Mary.

A Case of Total Allergy

The second case I would like to describe is one referred to me by her doctor who is a friend of mine. Below is the letter of referral received from my friend.

Dear Geoff,   Dated 7th January 1983

Re: Helen Carter,

Difficult to know what to say about Helen except she is a nice girl who I like very much and can't help to organise herself a bit better. Mother would like to think her problems are all allergy based, so would Helen. Her consultant physician and I feel sure that her troubles are largely psychological.

She has two brothers.

Hypnotherapy is the way Helen chose to get better I think—I suspect she may think this is something someone else will do for her. She has backed away from a psychological explanation in the past, as is clear from the literature on Helen,

Yours sincerely,
Helen's doctor.

Helen's date of birth 20th August 1958.

The following are letters enclosed with the letter above showing history going back as far as 1971.

I shall shorten these letters to show only that which seems relevant.

Letter from a consultant psychiatrist to Helen's doctor.

I saw Helen who is 13 years old first without her mother and then with Mrs Carter.

As I am sure you know Helen has been seeing 'visions' of her grandfather who died some twelve years ago. She has also been preoccupied with thoughts of death and losing her parents. She has few friends and is terribly shy and frightened of people.

There do not appear to have been any particular traumatic events in her life.

Her school experiences have been most unfortunate as at the previous day school she was unable to mix well and was allegedly bullied and treated unfairly even by members of the staff.

Helen is a thin, rather plain girl who looks younger than her age. She is very serious and appeared intelligent but having a strange manner as if she had already passed through her childhood and had not the normal emotional reactions of a young girl.

The next letter is from another psychiatrist to another doctor who was then treating Helen. This letter is Dated 9th May 1978.

Helen presented with a history of difficulty in mixing with strangers and meeting people since late childhood.

She has hardly any friends, and as she has grown up she has become more and more introverted, and withdrawn. Apparently she used to be "picked on" at school by even her close friends. She admits feeling like "a fish out of water." She is finding life more and more difficult to cope with, and is generally apprehensive so that she is unable to relax, sleeps poorly and gets depressed at times.

I do not think any tablets by themselves are going to be very helpful for Helen. I think she probably needs some behavioural modification to get over her undue fears and phobias. She has been advised to see our clinical psychologist as soon as possible.

17th August, 1978.

Helen is seen again by another psychologist who indicates that her lack of motivation to involve herself in therapy, suggests little progress will be made.

26th October, 1979.

She is seen by another consultant psychiatrist. Helen is complaining of depression and of sleeping fitfully owing to nightmares. She is scared of going into libraries, shops, public houses and cinemas, of meeting people and of travelling in trains and buses. She had experienced some boyfriend trouble, when one of her young men didn't reciprocate her feelings and another became psychologically disturbed.

The psychiatrist felt that Helen didn't relish the idea of

seeing another psychologist so he prescribed clomipramine. **(Anti Depressant.)**

22nd November, 1979.

Helen is seen by a consultant neurologist whose report is as follows;—

I note Helen has a problem with passing water, blurring of vision and now inability to walk.

On examination I found absolutely no focal neurological signs. There is normal power in the legs when she is tested lying in her bed but the moment she stands she collapses and then can be dragged along walking pigeon-toed. I have said to her very clearly that there is no disorder affecting the nervous system.

2nd January, 1980.

She goes back to the consultant psychiatrist who she saw previously. His report states:—

She is now walking normally but is histrionically depressed, complained of lassitude, anorexia, weeping and impaired concentration.

The consultant felt that Helen's mother's rather over possessiveness may be contributing to Helen's neurotic behavious, and suggested that she should be admitted to hospital. After her admission her parents felt the hospital environment upset Helen and she was eventually discharged with a full programme worked out by the senior clinical psychologist. It included social skills, vocational guidance, family therapy and in vivo desensitization for her agoraphobia.

19th August, 1980.

She is seen privately by a consultant psychologist whose report states:—

Helen's problems have been well described by the psychiatrists who have seen her in the past, though they have only hinted at the key role her parents have played in the origin and maintenance of her difficulty, emotional dependency about which she feels very ambivalent, and occasional episodes of acting out her frustrations with psychosomatic symptoms and tantrums.

He encouraged her to take a residential vocational course to get her away from her family which he thought would do her good.

13th February, 1981.

Helen visits yet another psychiatrist who states:—

She co-operated well at her interview and appeared a pleasant, intelligent and articulate young woman. Her main current problems were then a fluctuating mood state with periods of well-being and periods of functional paralysis. She experiences irrational panic feelings, impaired concentration, feelings of guilt, fluctuating appetite with anorexic periods and binge eating, sleep disturbances and behavioural outbursts in which she destroys objects including her own work.

She appears to be a young woman who is handicapped by her own extreme sensitivity and many of her present symtoms could be part of an atypical unresolved depression.

He suggests mono-amine oxidase inhibitors. **(Another Anti Depressant.)**

5th May, 1982.

Helen visits another psychologist who is a specialist in allergies. He feels that some of her problems stem from the fact that she seems to be allergic to a large number of perfectly normal things. He goes on to state that he feels this is not Helen's only problem. It is generally thought that both Helen and her mother would like to think that her problem is largely one of allergy.

I first saw Helen in January 1983. I asked her to write how she was and what she wanted to be. I also asked her mother if she could give me any information on Helen's birth and her early life. It seemed that the depression, anorexia, agoraphobia and claustrophobia may well be all First Line reactions to trauma at birth. On meeting Helen and her mother for the first time I was very agreeably surprised.

Helen's mother was a very charming and caring lady, not a bit like the description I had been led to believe from the notes I had received. Helen herself was an attractive, charming young lady, a little bit on the shy side, or perhaps a little reserved, but was that any wonder, after all the treatment she had received. She would obviously be anchored to failure. See below for her written description of how she was when I first saw her, by which time she was 24 years of age.

"HOW I AM.

I can't cope with stress—I panic and get blocked when I need to think or want to think—I feel unable to cope with normal life and be independent. I get so panicky and muddled and depressed if I think I'm proving myself or am self-conscious. Almost always amongst people or trying something new I can't cope. I hate myself, I feel ugly and weak and ashamed and guilty and worthless. I think people look down on me and I can't show them my best. It's humiliating to be seen as I am now, and it's taken a lot of will power and switching off to go anywhere or do anything with people, even my closest friends. I'm on the defensive having not been well with allergies, people don't understand and I think they think me over-sheltered and spoilt and lazy. I wonder if that's all that's wrong myself, I have put on a lot of weight in the past year and a half and people think I look well, so I feel guilty and ashamed. Deep down I know why I'm like this, but what people think makes me waver with guilt. I can't go to work or to college or even work hard on my own at home. I feel so ashamed I hide from people. I can't take their opinions, I can't explain, I'm jealous of them being able to eat what they want and being able to live too! I hate myself for the way I look and because I can't do anything am unable to cope and am so dependant on Mum, and insecure.

I'm scared of travelling, of driving, or going on buses or trains or planes etc., of going anywhere or being alone, of being scared of doing things badly or wrong, of being rejected. I always compare myself unfavourably with other people. I can't concentrate on anything. Television is my only means of escape from my guilt and self-hatred and dreams.

I can't face the empty days, afraid of wanting to eat, so I get up as near to midday as I can. At my worst I sit and watch television and eat all afternoon and evening and go to sleep about 3.00 in the morning. At my best I may work at my patchwork, even built a pot, knit, read or write, go for a walk, sometimes go to town with Mum. I don't feel safe without Mum. I help Mum about the house with a bit of cooking. I sometimes see two friends who have seen me when I was awful. At times I'm too ashamed to see even them.

I feel guilty, insecure, dissatisfied with myself—very unsure of myself now and afraid of the future. I disgust myself.

I'm restricted by my allergies, and even more by fear. I feel outside everything, unable to fit in, or join in. I'm so tired practically all the time, lethargic and negative. I feel incapable of ever coping, and can't distinguish the degrees that change from week to week of my capability. I'm afraid to even work at my pots at home, I can't bear to draw, it makes me too unhappy now.

I eat compulsively a lot of the time, am always thinking of food, afraid of it, what it does to me. I hate myself for wanting to eat the things that make me ill, when I'm so feeble even at the best of times, and fat. When things go wrong, I have to eat. When I want to do things and can't, I eat. When I want to avoid eating much, I eat and can think of nothing else. I can't join in when others drink, eat and are merry!

I can't concentrate consciously—I panic and lose my temper or go blank or go inside myself. All I can think of is wanting to be well and normal and not lonely. I tend to want to be what I think people want me to be, what will make me wanted. I'm full of conflict about myself. When with people, I'm so nervous and awkward, I don't feel a person, just an existence, and I feel disliked or boring. The only thing I can talk about is Art/craft, which I love.

Then I talk too much, nervously, and hate myself after. Whether I talk or not, am friendly or not, I hate myself. I'm so extremely self conscious, nearly all the time, and critical. I'm nervous in everything I do, even eating! I function best when I'm able to keep busy but am just with Mum or on my own.

I'm two stones overweight, my periods cause havoc, and my allergies lose control a bit as the period is due. I become more allergic and compulsive about food and lose ground. It is getting better with time and with the supra cortex injections I have had for the past five months and will have till September 84.

When I can stick to my diet, things are much easier and more enjoyable. According to my period, it's harder at times than others. Just before the period comes, from when it was due is too difficult and I have to eat more fruit and nuts, which help, but I put on weight again. Lately I haven't had to wait quite so long from the time it's due to its arrival and my weight has just gone up and down four or five pounds. That's better, but I want to lose weight! During those bad times I lose sight of all the positive, lose myself; hide, and am most negative. Now I don't eat anything bad, I'm scared to. I do eat the half-way bad things, but as time goes by, I realise more clearly what I can cope with and what I mustn't chance. I hope that as that happens, and as my periods begin to come on time and regularly, I may begin to slowly gain ground little by little at a time each month.

I cry very easily, at times, for no clear reason. Things remind me of feelings. I feel distant from people even at my best, and I think it shows that I don't belong or fit.

I think about death most days—and time going away, past, present and future.

I can't support myself financially or look after myself or stand up for myself. I can't remember what I think and feel, or feel that what I think and feel is as valid as anyone else. I can't believe in myself—I'm lethargic and negative. When I'm clear, I'm a lot less lethargic and negative, but never for long enough and the struggle becomes too big again for a time.

I can't sleep at night, nor get up the next day. Mostly I can't face a whole day, because I can't fill it, and because I eat.

HOW I WANT TO BE.

I want to be able to live and control my allergies, not let them get in the way of everything. I want to feel well. I want to be able to work hard at making pottery and patchwork quilts and to be able to exhibit and sell them and earn enough to be independent through them. I want to be calm about food, to accept my restricted diet, and to be able to lose two stones and then keep my weight under control and steady. I want to be able to be with friends and to make new friends. I wish I could accept myself, believe in myself and stop hating myself and wanting to hide. I want to be relaxed, calm, confident, receptive, able to cope, not to be afraid of everything and not be negative. I want to be able to think, be creative, able to use my brain without panic of failure. I want to feel strong and healthy. I want to be able to take responsibility, to trust myself, to trust people. I want to be able to have fun, to stop being so self-conscious. I want to be able to join in and communicate easily. I want all the depressing ugly thoughts to leave so there's room for positive useful creative thoughts. I want to have the strength and faith to try and work at the things I want, and to stop judging myself. I want confidence to do and enjoy the things I want to do, and forget about failure, opinions, right and wrong, time going by, death. . .

I want to be able to cope with fear and anger and nasties like that. I want to be able to be myself, and to be balanced, secure and steady. I want to stop thinking about Me, Me, Me all the time. I want to be able to learn, to read, see and absorb and understand and remember. I want to feel lively and positive, have courage, I want to be able to travel. I want to be able to withstand criticism, disappointment, wrong and fear. I want to stop getting at myself, comparing myself with other people, being jealous and insecure.

I want to be able to relax and forget about food. I want to be able to get up in the morning and be awake the whole day, and want to sleep again before midnight".

Helen's Mother's report

[1] I had a bad flu, with a very severe high temperature during the pregnancy.

[2] At eight months in my pregnancy I had a very bad migraine, with nausea, double vision, and very severe headache.

[3] The doctors told me that, although I had an anaesthetic during the last stage of birth, I screamed very loudly all the time.

[4] Although Helen was only 5lbs. 8oz. when she was born I still had to have stitches. Apparently it was quite a difficult birth.

[5] At three months Helen got a bad cold which left her with bronchial asthma for some time.

[6] She couldn't suckle. **(After a wipe out she probably wouldn't.)**

[7] When Helen was five she was afraid of crowds. (At her aunt and uncle's wedding reception.)

[8] She hated school, and had difficulties right from the start. I was quite surprised at this. It got worse as she got older, and some of the teachers seemed to really have it in for her. They made it very difficult for her and seemed to hate Helen.

[9] There was no jealousy when her brothers were born, but some jealous feelings seemed to develop later.

[10] Helen went to boarding school when she was 12-13. She wasn't happy there either.

[11] Helen hated going to parties, she wouldn't take her coat off. She couldn't stand noise and shouting. She said she felt ugly and wanted to get away from the noise. She has always seemed afraid of loud noises, even singing.

[12] She seems to panic if I am not well, and be afraid of my dying".

I did a Spiegel's capacity test with Helen and much to my surprise I found her to have a high hypnotic capacity, quite unlike Mary the previous patient in this chapter. This meant that, again unlike Mary, I should be able to use hypnosis reasonably efficiently with Helen. I decided that Helen's depression and self hatred were the first thing I should try and work on. I also asked her to keep a diary of how she felt from day to day. I also tested for O.B.D. as in Mary's case, and found as in Mary's case, Helen's reflexes were absent. I showed Helen the same set of exercises, and asked her to do these every day for twelve weeks.

With Helen in the hypnotic state I told her about the marathon she had won to be here, so she had asked to be here. I explained the journey of life and that she had just as much right as anyone else to be here, and make it to that higher plane. I taught her to enter the hypnotic state herself and to do all the exercises at the end of chapter 1. These exercises are to give her some anchor primal feelings to sustain her while we do the rest of her treatment. I repeated this treatment on several occasions until she began to feel a little better. Her day to day reports were full of negative thoughts, like "I don't know how I am going to get through today". I pointed out that with thoughts like that she was programming herself to have a bad day. Each week I went through her report and rubbed out the negative thoughts and replaced them with a more positive outlook. I gave her back her reports each week so that she could see how she was programming herself to make life difficult.

The following is one of her reports after she had had a little treatment.

"Why self inflict black thoughts?—, how can I be rid of them, other than squashing them. Why are they there at all? Isn't it more that I let myself feel bad rather than making myself bad. **(No you programme yourself to feel bad. You have learned to do that over the years when you** *were small, and you are still doing it to yourself.)*

Is it to do with hating myself and therefore with birth? *(Yes partly with birth and partly with your negative school experiences. They taught you to hate yourself.)*

This week.—better mentally. Tired and difficulty in breathing,—less terrified of losing my mind now. I'm not thinking about it all the time, I've a little more confidence now. I am beginning to do a little more, gradually—made two pots, drove the car, did a little drawing, went to see a ballet, beginning to read again, sticking better to very strict diet, all this week. Realising that I can do these things I want to if I believe in myself. Having difficulty in "loving myself!" Just forgetting myself helps. I avoid thoughts that lead me back to myself, or wanting independence, comparing myself and feeling jealous of people with the strength to live a full active sociable life. I feel such a boring drudge and ashamed of being a scaredy cat who does very little. *(There you go again knocking yourself.)* Even when I can work harder, I'll be working on my own, I can't imagine coping yet. I'm still afraid of what people will think of me, and want to avoid people for that, because I'm fat and boring. *(There you go again knocking yourself and programming yourself to be afraid of people. You can't know what people are thinking so don't imagine the worst.)*

Still it won't be for much longer, I'm sticking to my diet and very slowly losing weight, and I'm beginning to do a bit more too. It's building up and I'm doing five minutes every day, and consciously blocking negative thoughts and encouraging positive attitudes. *(Good! keep it up and do your exercises for two minutes every two to three hours until you feel much better.)*

Awful thoughts.—The future looks so bleak. *(It is what you make it, and you are programming it to be bad by the way you are thinking.)* Seeing people, I'm always afraid. *(You make yourself afraid, so stop. Once again programming yourself negatively.)* I'll never be able to cope, or make my pots and quilts as well as I want to. *(No you won't as long as you keep telling yourself that.)* I'm afraid of losing control, of rejection, of being alone, of being stupid, of being unable to relax and live. *(So long as you keep being afraid of those things, you programming yourself to feel them.)*

I make imaginary scenes of conversations in my head and I can't cope, or I'm horrid and useless, or alone, whether I am or not, and I imagine losing the people I love. *(Then stop doing that, and stop frightening yourself with imaginations.)*

I try to relax and imagine myself relaxed and able to cope, but worries get the upper hand. When I get too worried I don't want anything except to be alone and away from people.

So long as I don't think those thoughts, and I think only positive features, life seems less impossible, and my confidence grows. *(Then don't think negatively and be positive.)*"

On her next visit I had her think of three good things about herself. I had some difficulty getting her to admit that there were three good things about her, but in the end she could think of them easily. In an altered state of hypnosis I had her review those three good things and indulge herself in them, so that she could feel something good about herself. I had her repeat this exercise with herself every two or three hours until she could feel good about herself.

At this stage I did some 'Ideo Motor' questioning of her unconscious mind. At her birth, when her mother was screaming, her unconscious mind thought that somehow she was responsible for that, and in some way she was killing her mother. That's why she was so afraid of her mother dying. Her unconscious mind would have then succeeded in killing her. Her mother was present when we were doing this, and I had her mother tell Helen she would go through it all over again to have such a lovely daughter. I explained that as she had thought she nearly killed her mother she thought she wasn't a very nice person, but that had never actually happened so I reframed that thought. She has to know she didn't even try to kill her mother. She was very afraid of her mother's screaming so that was the start of her being afraid of loud noises, so I reframed noises, by making her see that it is one thing if someone is murdering someone else, but it is different if the noise is just a noise. In any case she had not been killing her mother so she need no longer be afraid of noises. As she had thought she had nearly killed her mother she felt very guilty, but as this had never really happened she needn't feel guilty any more. I reframed her guilt by making her see she was really a very caring person, where other people were concerned, and she could begin to care for herself. **(A start to make her love herself.)**

I reframed her thought that people didn't like her by making her see that this was a projection onto them of her own thought of not liking herself, and many of her friends did like her. They wouldn't keep coming back to see her if they didn't like her, and they did enjoy coming to see her so they must like her. Perhaps their liking her was more accurate estimation, of how she was, than her own feeling about herself.

We did some more work on these lines with my reframing her negative feelings, and Helen reinforcing that for herself afterwards, with auto hypnosis.

I received the following letter from Helen dated January 18th 1984.

Dear Mr. Graham,

With the usual ups and downs, I'm sure the improvement is building up. I still want to write my diaries, feel lost without them they help a lot, and I thought I'd send them to you before I come, but I hope it's not putting you out too much. I'm so forgetful and messy-minded I'll forget everything or distort it. **(Still knocking herself, and apologising for herself, so she hasn't learned to love herself yet.)** I think that what I'm wanting to work at now is being generally relaxed. Even now when times are definitely better and I'm coping more positively, I rarely relax, and it's very tiring. Well It's such a waste of time! **(It's good to get annoyed when you realise you are doing something you don't want to do, it helps you to make the change.)**

I hope you had a good Christmas and that the garden is not going to be too troubled by the snow. It's so beautiful here today, sunny and frosty. I'm doing the old housewife act at the moment! so I'm not getting much of my own stuff done. At least I'm not depressed now, that's a big relief. My mind is with my work even if I'm not doing it in practice, thinking and working things out is as important as doing things.
I will see you a week today. I look forward to it.
                Lots of love,
                Helen.

I worked on the fact that she was a grown woman now and not a young girl so she could learn to be adult with adult thoughts and feelings. I also reframed her courage, and self image again, all the time giving her a more accurate picture of herself.
On the 21st August 1984 I received the following letter from Helen.

"Dear Mr. Graham,
I'm just getting over the flu at the moment, back on my feet and down to work again thank goodness. I'm sorry I haven't been in touch for a while. I've been trying to decide what to do, and I think now I have decided to stop coming over to see you. I'm coping so much better, month by month, and I feel able to propel myself in the direction that's best for me, under my own steam. It's not that there are no downs, it's that I can see through them and they're more healthy, less destructive, and best of all the future isn't so frightening and dreadful. I even look forward nowadays. Some very good friends have asked me to go to India with them some time! They have parents living in the mountains in the north. I'm so excited, it's somewhere I'd really love to go once in my life. I have an open invitation, but mustn't leave it too long because of the situation there. What better incentive could I have, and what better timing? I'm hoping to go in the autumn next year maybe.

My pots are going on well, a slow but definite development with each firing. At the moment I'm doing only earthenware, (the red clay) and firing the pots once in the electric kiln, to 1000 degrees, then firing them in sawdust in an incinerator overnight, and the clay becomes beautifully marked by the carbon. It's the kind of work I enjoy most, but am not giving up on glazes. I made a little set of coffee cups and saucers, my first, and gave half to one of my friends and the other to another.

She goes on to say what she is doing with her pottery and then:

"So, all being well, very soon, life should be more mobile and sociable for me, which I do want however tentative I'm feeling about each step towards people! It's the "wanting" that's just beating the "being frightened" at long last! I want to learn, I want to write and draw and paint and to make pots and patchwork and I want to be with people, more and more, and the fear is dying down. I suppose as my attitude towards myself relaxes and calms down.

As I leave myself alone, I can force my mind to do what I want to do. It's happening slowly, but I can see it and appreciate it now, and that makes patience and positiveness easier. I'm much stronger. I don't know what I can do exactly, if I can be a good potter, writer, etc. but I want to do this work more than anything, as well as I can.

So if it is all right with you, can I keep in touch writing to you, and the odd phone call? I want to thank you very much.

Love,
Helen".

Helen's life had not gone smoothly but she is still coping, in spite of her involvement with a disturbed young man, and she is still developing. I have seen her again recently and we are working on making her more independent and responsible for herself. She is looking much more like a grown lady than the little girl who first came to see me (in spite of the fact she was 24 years old when she first came.)

Miracles Happen Only Rarely

My third and last case in this book is about a man who I shall call Phillip. Phillip came to see me because he was falling down about six times a day. He had been falling down for about ten years before coming to see me. He didn't know when it would happen but he knew for certain that it would happen about six times every day. He said it was getting very difficult as he didn't know when it would happen, and he was beginning to not go out. He said "I may be just going into a pub for a drink and I may fall down, and the landlord would tell me to leave, thinking I was already drunk". Phillip had been privately to the Nuffield Hospital where he had been wired up and tested for everything. The Nuffield has a very good reputation for its standard of excellence. They tested him for faulty brain waves, for blood flow to the brain, for potassium levels in his blood and everything else you can think of. He was there for a whole day and fell down about six times while wired up, but still they could find nothing organically wrong.

They didn't ask him a very important question, which is, *"If you fall down about six times a day, and have been doing so for the last ten years, how many times have you seriously hurt yourself?"* His answer was "never". So I told him he must be choosing where he falls down. You can't fall down six times a day for ten years and never hurt yourself unless you choose where you fall down. He obviously was choosing where, unconsciously, as he wasn't aware of making a choice, but nevertheless he must be choosing. He had to admit it sounded right, after he had thought about it. He asked me why was he doing it? Obviously I didn't know, I had only just met him, so I decided to do a capacity test to see if I could use hypnosis to find out.

I did a modified 'Spiegel' capacity test which ended up with the patient in a trance and his hand on his shoulder. I told him that his shoulder may want to keep his hand there, even though he may want to remove it. His shoulder may want to keep it there so much that even if he tried to remove it the harder he tried to remove it the harder his shoulder may keep it there. I told him that I would now wake him up but his shoulder may still keep his hand there even though he was wide awake. I wanted to test him for post hypnotic suggestion just in case I wanted to use it in his therapy. I woke him from trance and found him to have a very high capacity indeed. Although he was wide awake he was quite unable to move his hand from his shoulder, thus responding very well to my post hypnotic suggestion. I asked him why he felt he couldn't move his hand away? He didn't know, so I explained that he was doing just that to his legs when he fell down. He said he understood.

I re-hypnotised him and said I would remove the suggestion if he would stop falling down. He agreed readily. I taught him auto hypnosis and told him to do the split screen with himself falling down on one side, and himself being perfectly steady and not falling down on the other side, and to tell his mind which one he wanted to be. His hour was up so I brought him out of trance and as I was just about to go to America I said I would ring him up as soon as I returned.

While in America as I was attending a large clinical hypnosis meeting, I asked around to see if anyone had treated a case like Phillip. I eventually found one doctor who had had about five cases like Phillip. The doctor said all you have to do is find out from their unconscious mind why they are falling down and they stop falling down. I could hardly wait until I returned, and immediately phoned Phillip and made him another appointment to see him.

When he came in I explained that I had found another doctor who had had five cases like him and the doctor said all we had to do was find out why his unconscious mind was making him fall down and he would stop falling down. Phillip said "Hang on a bit. I haven't fallen down since I last saw you." This was some four weeks previously. I asked him *Do you mean to tell me you haven't fallen down for four weeks?"*

"That's right."

"Have you ever not fallen down for four weeks since you started to fall down?"

"No."

He has not fallen down since his first visit, which was some three years ago, and I never did find out why his unconscious mind made him fall down in the first place. I can say, that whatever the reason was in the past, it is certainly no longer valid, otherwise he would not have been able to give up that behaviour so readily.

CHAPTER 6
Conclusions

It is impossible for any parent to be there, to attend to every need of their child for twenty-four hours a day, so sooner or later the child is going to hurt. When that happens the natural defence is first to pretend it is not happening. To do this, the child stops feeling the hurt by denial. If it repeatedly denies something it learns not to feel. Neurosis is a faulty perception on the 'feeling' side of the brain (right hemisphere in right handed people, or the non-dominant side of the brain. Because of the cross over in the brain, the non-dominant side is the same side as our dominant eye, hand and foot; the one we aim with, write with, and kick a ball with). They learn to think one thing and feel another. The confusion leads to the production of fear, anxiety, anger or guilt. This confusion and heightened state of negative emotion causes the mind to try to help the person to achieve a state of homeostasis or balanced comfort, by a behaviour that worked in the past. A regressive behaviour that once helped in one set of circumstances doesn't necessarily help in a new situation, and may even make it worse. The way the mind is trying to help, in these difficult situations, frequently becomes the problem. So neurotic behaviour is a regressive behaviour to a more child-like defence, to anxiety, etc. which doesn't help the problem and may even make it worse.

There are only two types of people, the happy neurotic, and the unhappy one. Everybody is neurotic. It is impossible to go on the journey through life without being hurt. The happy neurotic has some options in life, the unhappy one has none. Love is the best cure for hurt, therefore the cure for neurosis is love. It is hoped that both our parents love each other and love us, so that we may grow up in a safe and secure environment and become a happy neurotic with options in life.

As I said earlier it is impossible not to get hurt at some time or other. Parents fail to be loving for a number of reasons and succeed in screwing up their children, because of their own unfelt pain. They may have married for the wrong reasons, and found out they are not suited, or more commonly some negative anchor is forcing them to reject each other. A common example of this is where one partner is feeling bad or low for one reason or another, when the second partner comes on the scene they cuddle each other. This may, however, not solve the negative feeling and may anchor feeling bad to the act of cuddling. The next time they cuddle even if they are both feeling good, because of the negative anchor, the partner who was feeling bad the first time begins to feel bad again. This reinforces the negative anchor. Pretty soon the one who feels bad doesn't want to cuddle any more because it makes them feel bad. The other one feels rejected and says "you don't love me any more". This just annoys the first one because it doesn't fit with how they feel and makes them feel guilty for not cuddling, but they can't tell their partner that cuddling them makes them feel bad. They also don't know why it should have that effect. Very quickly the whole thing blows up totally out of proportion and we have two parents at loggerheads with each other for no reason, except a negative anchor, that neither has recognised, each blaming the other, and neither having the necessary skill to do anything about it. I believe more marriages are on the rocks for something simple like that than have real major problems.

Their children may trigger off their own unfelt pain from their own childhood; thus they have to reject the child or feel pain. Hence "the sins of the father visit the children until the seventh generation." What a great shame it is that most of us only learn what we should have done for our children when we are too old either to have them, or be bothered with them. I have frequently heard patients say "my parents never showed me any love but they are very good with the grandchildren."

If our parent couldn't be what we needed when we were

young, the only cure is for us to become the parent we never had.

If we look at chapters 2, 3 and 4 we can see that it is possible to tell from the symptoms and the history and the way of telling it all, when we learned a particular piece of behaviour. This gives us a clue about when a trauma may have occurred and can save a lot of time when we are trying to pinpoint that time in the patient's personal history.

There are certain essential criteria in the business of psychotherapy. The first is to treat people not symptoms. In my opinion it is far too common to see patients labelled as say depressives, or obese and then treat a case of depression, or obesity. Everyone is unique; no two people will experience the world and the things in it, in exactly the same way, and their responses may be quite different. If you treat every fat person as a case of obesity it's likely you will have a large number of failures. The purpose of psychotherapy is to help someone with disturbed thoughts, feelings and actions which reduce the patient's options in life, to find more options and thereby reduce those disturbances and encourage more desirable behaviour.

The second essential criterion for the patient and therapist is for them both to be aware of the patient's difficulties and to have some idea of what they are trying to achieve with the therapy. It is no good the therapist trying to tell the patient what the patient should do, be or feel. No therapist has the right to tell anyone what they should do, be or feel. As the patient is unique, no therapist can know what is best for them. There are far too many 'do gooders' in the world already.

It is most important that the patient picks the right therapist for them. No therapist can treat everyone. The right therapist should be comparatively stable with not too many hang-ups, or at least understand his own hang-ups. I have seen therapists unconsciously treat themselves through the patient without even realising it, because they were unaware of their own hang-ups. This to me is entirely dishonest as the patient is the one who is paying. Bad therapists get therapy a bad name, it is often not the therapy that is no use, but the therapist. Unfortunately many people with severe hang-ups are often attracted to become therapists, but if their hang-ups are unresolved they make bad therapists. Fully treated therapists are often very good as they have a good understanding of what the patient is going through, having been 'there' themselves.

The therapist should be aware of the patient's problem, and demonstrate that he understands it properly. Therapists owe it, both to their patients and themselves, to feel that they are capable of helping the patient. If they don't feel this, they shouldn't take the patient for treatment. If the therapist doesn't think that he and the patient can succeed they probably won't, and just end up getting everybody frustrated. Incidentally, if they try treatment and are unsuccessful and persevere with unsuccessful strategies, they only anchor the patient to failure. I have too often seen therapists who go on and on with the same treatment and get nowhere except in anchoring the patient to failure. If something doesn't work then for goodness sake do something else before the patient becomes negatively anchored. This is one of the dangers in Primal therapy, the patient becomes anchored to feeling pain. Often the therapist goes on with unsuccessful treatment because they themselves don't know what else to do. In this case they should refer the patient to someone more experienced, if they know of someone, or seek advice from other therapists who may have encountered similar cases.

The therapist must have, and show, some respect for the patient otherwise the patient will percieve this lack of respect and if they continue in therapy will begin to believe they are no good. That's why they need therapy in the first place, because their parents showed this lack of respect for them and they believed it. On a few occasions I have had requests from people to cure their inferiority complex. After a short while I have felt that they don't have a complex, they are just inferior. I have never continued with their therapy.

The object of the therapy is to allow the patient to see they have more choices in life and have assistance in thinking more positively about themselves, and eventually to be able to love themselves.

This is often done by encouraging the patient to release and express their pent-up feelings and emotions in a safe environment, established by the therapist's understanding and warmth towards the patient. A young lady who was having treatment for the first time with me began to get very agitated when I talked to her in a loud voice, so I talked a little louder. As she got more agitated she began to scream "I hate you, I have always hated you, all my life". I said *"That's funny, I have only just met you today. Who is that you have hated all your life?"* She burst into tears and said "my mother, she has always been terrible to me" so I had to teach her 'to be the parent she never had.'

The patient must try out their increased options by testing reality. They will never get better just listening to the therapist. The treatment should be designed to enable the patient to mature and become responsible for themselves, and be the parent they never had. All this will take time. Many patients often expect to go to a hypnotist and be hypnotised once and walk out cured. It doesn't happen that way, it often takes quite a long time. Unfortunately because of the time taken, psychotherapy is often very expensive, but what price is good health and happiness? Miracles happen only rarely.

The exercises in this book may seem to be blanket treatments for symptoms. It is essential when doing them, that you realise that full treatment entails treatment of the whole person, not just symptoms. They will, however, help you to make a start to become mature, and the rest will depend on whether you need professional assistance, or not, in fully becoming your own parent.

APPENDIX
The Exercises

EXERCISE 1.   Find a comfortable chair preferably with a high back which will support your head. Sit comfortably in the chair and rest your head on the back. Place your feet with your soles flat on the ground. At this point I always suggest that female patients remove their shoes. Ladies tend to take off their shoes when returning home after work, a shopping expedition, an evening out etc. and it is therefore a major aid to their relaxation. Place both your arms comfortably and lightly on each armrest of the chair; if there are no armrests on the chair, place one hand upon each knee. Do not fold your arms or clasp your hands, as both these behaviours are defensive. Look straight ahead of you then, without altering the position of your head, turn your eyes up to look towards your eyebrows. Turn them up as high as you can without moving your head. Keeping your eyes turned up close your eyes. (SPIEGEL'S EYEROLL INDUCTION) (1).

Now relax your eyes, let them become so relaxed, so heavy they feel they just won't open, and hang on to that feeling. Now let that feeling spread through the whole of your body. Let your body sink comfortably down into the chair. (ELMAN DEEPENING) (2).

While your body is sinking down into the chair turn your mind inward to look at your mind. (GEOFF GRAHAM & N. L. P.) Let your mind feel as if it can float. (SPIEGEL) (3).

While your body is sinking comfortably into the chair and your mind is pleasantly floating, turn your thoughts to something that gives you great pleasure and joy. Let yourself enjoy that feeling as much as you can. Hang on to that good feeling and imagine how good it would be to be wide awake with your eyes wide open with that good feeling. (GEOFF GRAHAM'S SCRAP BOOK) (4). Now open your eyes and be wide awake with that good feeling.

EXERCISE 2.   Before doing all these exercises it is better to enter that heightened state of concentration described in exercise 1, up to the part where you turn your mind inwards to look at your mind. While you are looking at your mind, contemplate that marathon you ran to be here and tell yourself that by winning that race YOU ASKED TO BE HERE.

EXERCISE 3.   While you are in that heightened state of consciousness and thinking about having asked to be here, remember that there is no-one on this earth for any other reason than winning a marathon. Therefore tell yourself, YOU HAVE JUST AS MUCH RIGHT AS ANY OTHER PERSON TO BE HERE.

EXERCISE 4.   By winning that marathon race you proved that you were the fittest of fifty million to survive, and you have the right to take the journey through life and win. So tell yourself, YOU CAN WIN AND BE A SUCCESS AND RAISE YOUR CONSCIOUSNESS TO THAT HIGHER PLANE.

EXERCISE 5.   Tell yourself YOU WILL WIN SO THAT YOU WON'T HAVE TO DO IT ALL OVER AGAIN, AND WILL BECOME RESPONSIBLE FOR YOURSELF.

EXERCISE 6.   YOU LIKE YOURSELF FOR WINNING A MARATHON AND YOU WILL LEARN TO LOVE YOURSELF.

EXERCISE 7.   While you are in that heightened state of concentration think about one or two of the good things about yourself, and celebrate those things by feeling good about them. It is essential you learn to celebrate things about yourself. At first you may have some difficulty in thinking good things about yourself because of a birth wipe out, but you must persevere until you can. Remember you must learn

THE EXERCISES

to love yourself so that others can, then you can feel secure because security is being loved.

EXERCISE 8. Migraine sufferers. While in an altered state, find and thank the part of the mind that enabled you to make your head smaller at birth by first decreasing your intracranial pressure at a time of stress, and then reflating that pressure afterwards, but respectfully remind it that when your skull is firmly united this altering of pressure is no mature way of responding to stress. There are much better ways of responding to, and handling stress. (For these ways see chapter 6.) Ask it to try one or two of the more mature ways and give it the option. If that way doesn't work try another until one does, and you have no need then to have migraine.

EXERCISE 9. Agoraphobics in an altered state must realise that the places in which they feel afraid are very different from the birth canal. After all, they did get out safely in the end. They do this by creating images of those places where they would normally want to get out of, and telling themselves that they will be able to get out quite easily when they need to, and until that time, they will enjoy where they are, and feel very safe there. You can create an image in many ways. You may be able to see it. If you can't, however, don't worry just think about it, and you will have a conceptual image. It is impossible to think about anything without forming some sort of image. Create that image in whichever way you normally think about things.

EXERCISE 10. Asthmatics in an altered state create images of their breathing tubes relaxing and allowing the air to flow in, and particularly out, freely and easily. They see themselves taking control of their breathing and it becomes easier in all circumstances. Also learn some of the stress reducing exercises in chapter 6.

EXERCISE 11. This exercise is for people suffering from guilt and a feeling of being a nuisance, or feeling they should not be here. People whose apologetic nature makes me call them 'Sorry-merchants'. In an altered state they must tell themselves that the purpose of life is to mature, otherwise they will just have to do it all over again. Have them create an image of being born, watching themselves experiencing that feeling of wipe out but reassuring themselves that every one concerned with the birth wants them to be alive, well, and get out easily. Have them reassure themselves that they did get out and it's over now and they need never feel like that again. They, and everyone else wanted them to be here, so there is no need to apologise.

EXERCISE 12.   If people haven't made a bond with a parent immediately following the birth, and have difficulty in looking people straight in the eyes without feeling uncomfortable, have them watch their own birth, and have them make eye to eye contact with themselves, as they are now, and themselves being born, while the adult self is thinking I love you and will help you to feel good.

This is the first step to becoming your own parent. (see chapter 5).

EXERCISE 13.   SPIEGEL'S SPLIT SCREEN.

First of all, use auto-hypnosis to enter a special state of heightened concentration. When you begin to feel your mind comfortably floating as if it were free, imagine a cinema, or television, screen, divided down the middle, on the wall in front of you. If you can see it, so much the better, but if you can't just think about it as a conceptual image. You don't have to see it for this technique to work. While you have the image of the screen on the other side of the room, see (either visually or conceptually) the behaviour you would like to change on one half of the screen. Now see the behaviour you would like to have to replace the unwanted one on the other side of the screen. Choose which behaviour you want and tell your mind. Having chosen, bring back from the screen the behaviour you would like, leaving the one you don't want on the other side of the room. Integrate the desired behaviour with your mind by thinking how good it would be to have

THE EXERCISES

that desired behaviour (see operant conditioning in the second chapter), and how you would feel doing it. (Teaching you to feel real feelings again). Integrate your mind with your body, open your eyes and go and adopt the desired behaviour.

EXERCISE 14.   IDEO-MOTOR FINGER RESPONSES.

When you are talking to someone in a perfectly normal state of consciousness, and you are asking them a question to which they answer "yes", watch their head. Ask them another question to which they will answer "yes" and watch their head again. Most people answering "yes" to a question will not only say "yes", but at the same time they will nod their head. Ask them without telling them, "what did they do when they answered the question" and most of them won't have a clue what they did, showing that the nod of the head is an unconscious answer. The same is true of a negative answer when they shake the head.

While people are talking, even in a normal state of consciousness, two parts of their mind are listening, paying attention and answering. The conscious mind is answering by verbally saying "yes" or "no" but at the same time the unconscious mind is also answering by nodding or shaking the head. This nodding or shaking the head is called an ideo-motor response. It is a response from the unconscious mind. We often set this up deliberately so that we can explore the unconscious mind. If we are being affected by something which happened to us long ago, we must have a memory of it somewhere within us; if this were not the case, it would not be affecting us now. This memory, however, is often long since forgotten consciously, but it is still in the unconscious somewhere. We can explore the unconscious mind in an altered state by asking the unconscious to answer our questions by lifting a finger of one of our hands, say the index finger of the left hand, or often it is better to let the unconscious mind choose which finger it will use. It can use one finger for "yes" and another for "no", in this way we can ask it yes or no questions. You can even have an "I don't know" finger, and an "I don't want to answer" finger, but I feel having too many alternatives often confuses the answer. We are much less used to lying with our finger so we may well get a more honest answer this way. It is not, however, infallible and the finger can lie. So we just ask our unconscious mind if it will answer in this way and if it will, will it please lift a "yes" finger. One finger should rise. Establish a "no" finger in the same way and if you get a response both times you should be able to ask it some more questions that may help you to have more options. It is not so easy to do this by yourself but if it is first done with a therapist many patients can do it by themselves. The skill is often in knowing what to ask it, and what to do about it when you get an answer.

EXERCISE 15. CREATING NEW RESOURCES FROM OLD.
In the case of my colleague, Alan, who was frightened to get up and ask a question at a professional meeting for fear of humiliation, I had him think of a time in the past when he wanted to show off, or was very brave. He had some difficulty in remembering an occasion, but eventually told me his mother reminded him of when they used to go to the beach. The particular beach they went to had a wall running along the edge. When Alan was small he would run along the wall and when he reached a high part, he would shout, "Mummy, Mummy look at me" and then jump onto the sand. The resource he was feeling at the time of shouting to his mummy had to be, "Aren't I clever?, I want you to see how clever I am and tell me". Wouldn't that be a good resource to feel at a meeting if he wanted to ask a question, and wouldn't it help him to overcome his fear if he could feel it?

I had Alan in an altered state review that scene on the beach while he shouted "Mummy! Mummy! look at me". While he was feeling as much of that scene as he could he was to rub his thumb over the tips of his fourth, middle and index fingers. The rubbing of his fingertips with his thumb is equivalent to Pavlov's bell. Feeling the scene is equivalent to Pavlov's feeding the dogs, so by doing that for about two to three minutes at a time, about five times a day, for twenty days he was creating a simple Pavlovian conditioned reflex of feeling, "Aren't I clever?, I want you to see how clever I am", to rubbing his fingertips. After that time he would be able to feel "Aren't I clever?, I want you to see how clever I am", by just rubbing his fingertips together. I feel it is a nice concept of having resources at your fingertips. So the next time he was at a meeting, and he wanted to ask a question, after he had created the reflex, all he had to do was to rub his fingertips together, and get up and ask away.

If you are afraid to do something then create a conditioned reflex to feeling brave from a time when you were actually brave, or stood up for someone or something. You can create a feeling of confidence from a time when you were happy and confident. All you need is a time in the past when you had a resource that would be useful now in the behaviour you would like to change, create the reflex, and go ahead with the new feeling from the past.

EXERCISE 16.   NEGOTIATING BETWEEN THE PARTS.
When there are two functions, both of which are necessary (but at different times) and these are interfering with each other, it is possible to help the situation and behaviour by negotiating between the two parts of the mind responsible for those two functions. See the example above, in sleeping and being awake. Another example is in concentration while working and relaxing afterwards, or learning to switch off.

Many people who have very demanding, busy, and exacting jobs find great difficulty in switching off, at weekends or evenings, without some form of drug etc. Commonly the drug thought to be the lesser of the evils is alcohol. Perhaps this is why there are so many alcoholics in the professions. Wouldn't it be much better to learn to switch off with our minds instead of alcohol, or whatever? To do that, all that is necessary is to enter an altered state of consciousness and go inside the mind and find the respective parts responsible first for concentration, then for relaxation. Thank both parts for their respective functions. Ask each to listen, pay attention, and be willing to negotiate. Set up an ideo-motor response for both parts in one or another of each index fingers (as in text of chapter 4). Negotiate first with one part then with the other and ask each to respond as in text of chapter 4. Having got a response from each, ask them to confirm their willingness to begin to help you in this new negotiated way, from right now, by coming together and touching, as a token of shaking hands on the deal, as our wonderful Irish friend put it. I always use what people come up with if it is a good idea.

EXERCISE 17.   FOR REACTIVE DEPRESSION.
First of all it is necessary to find out what is causing the depression, or which of the three reasons, mentioned in the text, is responsible for the negative feelings. The first question is "did you cry and feel really bad at the time?" If not, you possibly haven't felt it all, and need to. The second question is "do you miss not having the person around and will nothing, or no one, ever be able to replace your need for them?" If the answer is yes to both those questions then you have too great a dependence on someone else and need to become your own parent. The third question is "do you feel bad that they are no longer here and you won't ever be able to tell them how much you loved them?" If the answer is yes, you are suffering from guilt. You may be suffering from one, two, or all three of these reasons.

If you haven't felt the grief then it is probably better to find a therapist to help you to do that by talking about it openly, while the therapist encourages you to feel what you are talking about, and at the same time provides the necessary support while you are doing so. Entering an altered state will often facilitate the release of repressed feelings, or hyperventilating will do the same. Either of these techniques should be done with the support of a good therapist, in case you get into a feeling that you can't handle on your own.

If you are overdependent on the lost one, you need to become the parent you never had. It may be the lost one is not your parent, but overdependence is always a child-parent relationship, and you are using a parent substitute. Remember the purpose of life is to mature and become responsible for yourself. Most of the exercises in this book are designed to help you become the parent you never had, and mature, and become responsible for yourself.

It may be useful for you to remember that the good experiences you had with the lost one can't be taken away from you by their not being here. An experience is an experience that you have had, and can't be taken away, because you have already had it. It is your experience for the rest of your life. You may not be able to repeat the experience, but that which you have had can't be taken away from you. I am sure your loved one would like to live on in your memory as a good experience, and not as a sad feeling. In exactly the same way, I'm sure when you go, you would like your loved ones to remember you with the good experiences you have had together, and not with bad feelings.

If you feel bad, and guilty, because you never told your lost one how much you really loved them, remember that to feel bad about them when they have gone is like rubbing salt into the wound. You can show them how much you really love them by feeling really good about the good things about them, and using those good things to sustain you for the rest of your life. So tell yourself all the good things you know about your lost one, in an altered state, and feel really good that you had such a good store of good experiences with them. This way you can show the world how much you loved them.

EXERCISE 18. Still in an altered state of consciousness I asked Frank to review the first of the hurtful episodes he had spoken about earlier, as if it were a film. While he was watching himself as a child, (his 'child's mind'), he was to go to his "child self", and tell that little boy that he loved him. That he understands him. That he will help him to grow up. That his 'child self' need never feel so alone or hurt again. That he can be anything he really wants, and he doesn't need to fail to win because he (his 'adult mind') will help his 'child self'. We then went through each of the traumas Frank had remembered in the altered state, asking his 'adult mind' to comfort and encourage the child Frank in each case as above. When we finished, we asked his unconscious mind to indicate with an ideo-motor finger response if there were any more occasions he felt alone, or afraid, hurt and unloved. Of course, there were others which we had to work through. I then worked on reframing Frank's defences, by showing him that there were much better ways to defend himself as an adult, than losing, and it would be much easier if he was able to concentrate for as long as necessary. I told him he could really beat his father by being successful.

EXERCISE 19.   In the hypnotic state, first find out from your unconscious mind what attention you needed and didn't get, then have yourself fantasize giving yourself that attention while you are holding your younger self. At the same time reassure your younger self that they need never feel so alone or afraid again because you will give them all the attention they need to grow up in a safe, secure and loving environment. Reassure your younger self that they needn't resort to desperate means (the symptoms produced to get attention by your 'child self'), or even the neurotic behaviour that they are making you carry out now, to get attention because you (the adult you) will help them (the child you) to find more adult ways of getting attention. Or better still to find ways of coping without needing attention (becoming responsible for self, the process of maturing, and the purpose of life).

EXERCISE 20.   In Tom's case, I had him enter the state of hypnosis (altered state of consciousness), and while relaxing, create an image of himself in a cinema, first of all with the screen blank. While he was looking at the blank screen, he was to take his mind to the row behind his body, thus watching his body in the row in front watching the screen. This way he couldn't feel his body in the row in front. He was then to watch himself, in the row in front, watching a film of his birth on the screen. With his mind he was to see his 'baby self' stuck, with his legs out, and everybody trying to get his head out safely. He was to take his mind to the screen, leaving his body back in the cinema watching his mind talking to his 'baby self'. His mind was to tell his 'baby self' that he knew his 'baby self' would get out safely because his mind was his 'baby self' from the future. His mind was also to tell his 'baby self' that everybody involved wanted to help him get out safely and no-one wanted to hurt him, let alone pull his head off. His mind was to tell his 'baby self' that his mother wanted him alive and well and she loved him very much, but during the birth she couldn't tell him that, so Tom must now tell him. His 'adult' mind was to use all its power of persuasion to convince his 'baby self' that all these things were true, and to help his 'baby self' get out feeling safe, loved and wanted. When his 'baby self' had got out believing these things, he was to tell it he loved it and then go back to the row behind his body in the cinema. He was then to go back into his body seeing his 'baby self' 'out', safe, and feeling loved by everybody. He was to repeat this exercise until he felt his 'baby self' believed him. It took quite a time before this happened, but when it did he no longer had any fear of having his head knocked off in places with people serving behind counters.

EXERCISE 21. In the case of migraine, have the patient dissociate their mind from their body and watch a film of their birth with their head stuck. Have their mind tell their 'baby self' that by decreasing their intra-cranial pressure they made it possible for them to get their head out more easily but they never need do that again unless they are being actually reborn. When they are 'out' have their mind tell their 'baby self' that the reflation helped them to restore the shape of their head, but they never need do that again especially when their cranial bones are fully united. Tell them that everyone loves them including yourself and they are wanted and no one was trying to get rid of them, or wipe them out. Tell them you will show them much more mature ways of dealing with stress (see chapter 6).

EXERCISE 22. Patients suffering from depression should see themselves stuck, in the birth canal, generally with the head through the arch and their shoulders stuck, unable to go forwards or backwards. Have their 'adult minds' tell their 'baby self' that the only defence in this situation is to stop feeling but that their 'adult mind' knows that they will get 'out' safely because their 'adult mind' is their 'baby self' from the future. Reassure them that everybody wants them 'out' and safe, and everybody loves them. Have their 'adult mind' see their 'baby self' get 'out' and persuade the 'baby self' that it is both safe and necessary to feel again. It is especially necessary to feel that they are 'out' and it is no longer unsafe to feel. In the future there will be much better defences, to situations in which they may feel stuck, than not feeling. To 'not feel' in future situations will just ensure that they are unable to do anything about the unpleasant positions they may find themselves in. Have them repeat this exercise until they begin to feel again, and their depression begins to lift. Then teach them new defences to stress. (See chapter 6.)

EXERCISE 23.   With patients suffering from Anorexia Nervosa, have them see themselves struggling to get 'out' and in the struggle getting the cord entangled. Have their adult mind see and persuade their 'baby self', that it is nobody's fault especially their 'friend and provider', the cord, or their mother. In any case have their 'baby mind' see that they do get 'out' safely and that in future they have no cause to reject the 'provider' (sustenance for themselves in the form of food) or 'mother' or blame either of them. They do not need to reject mother by killing themselves by not eating, as she was not guilty of trying to kill them. They do not need to be afraid of growing up and taking responsibility because they did ask to be here by winning a marathon and the purpose of being here is to mature. It is no use fighting the purpose of life because you can't win. If you die you just have to do it all over again so you may as well find a way of enjoying the journey and making it to that higher plane this time round. Have them repeat this exercise until they can respond to all the other treatment, some of which is described in chapter 2. This exercise will give them the parent (the need to mature and become responsible) they thought quite wrongly they didn't have at birth.

EXERCISE 24.   To bond with yourself enter the hypnotic state and watch a film of yourself being born. Immediately you are born ('out') take your 'adult mind' to your 'baby self' and hold your 'baby self' lovingly while your 'adult mind' looks lovingly into your 'baby self's' eyes. When you can see that loving look returned by your 'baby self' the bond has been established and the patient will find it much easier to look people in the eyes without feeling uncomfortable. Repeat this exercise until you have no difficulty in looking people straight in the eyes.

EXERCISE 25.   After entering hypnosis, access a peaceful relaxing scene of your own choice. Access all the feelings connected to that scene and hold on to them. Now imagine how good it would be to be wide awake, performing whatever you have to do next with those good feelings. Then just open your eyes and carry on.

EXERCISE 26.   'Goal directed meditation with visualisation of your own stress meter.' After entering hypnosis concentrate on your breathing. Become particularly aware of each breath out you take. It is relaxing to breathe out. It is like letting go of a balloon that is blown up. The sides of the balloon collapse down and the tension in the wall disappears. Breathing out is the same. When you breathe out the tension in the lung lining disappears, your lungs collapse down and the air is pushed out. Your unconscious mind is aware of the reduction in tension so you feel relaxed. You 'feel' on the nondominant side of your brain, so you feel relaxed on the nondominant side with each exhalation. You think on the dominant side of your brain so if you think of the word 'calm' and what that means as you breathe out, you both think and feel relaxed. As explained in the 'think feel' theory chapter 2 in this book it is much more efficient if you both think and feel the same thing at the same time. So if you think "calm" every time you breathe out, you begin to reduce tension. This is goal directed meditation.

At the same time as you are co-ordinating your breathing out with thinking "calm" you can picture your own personal stress meter. Your stress meter can be any form of metering system that is comfortable to you, but for the sake of the description in this exercise, let us think of it like a parking meter. If you are feeling tense then you should access you meter with the penalty sign showing. Each breath out you take, while you are thinking "calm", is like putting another coin in the meter. Soon the penalty sign disappears and you feel more relaxed. If you go on co-ordinating your breathing with thinking "calm" the meter gets lower and lower, as you get more and more relaxed. Once you have lowered your tension, just like the parking meter, it doesn't immediately go up again. So if you practice this technique every few hours the penalty of feeling tense should not have to be paid, and you will become much more relaxed. Do this exercise three or four times a day for two minutes at a time.

EXERCISE 27.   Spiegel's split screen technique. In the hypnotic state, when you feel floating, access the split screen on the other side of the room. On one side see yourself tense and uptight. On the other side see yourself relaxed and calm, then tell yourself which one you want to be. Access all the feelings of the one you want to be, and bring them back from the screen leaving the 'you' you don't want on the other side of the room. Then imagine how good it will be to be doing whatever you are doing feeling like that. Open your eyes and be like that. Repeat the exercise every few hours, for two minutes at a time, until you feel well.

EXERCISE 28.   Ego strengthening. In the hypnotic state access the marathon you ran to be here. Tell yourself that you have as much right as anyone else to be here. Tell yourself that you have as much right to be as relaxed as anyone else here. Access how relaxed that can be, then open your eyes and be that relaxed. Repeat the exercise every few hours until you feel comfortable.

EXERCISE 29.   Reframing. In the hypnotic state access that part of the mind that is making you tense, in an attempt to help you cope with a situation. Ask it, when it is listening, paying attention, and willing to negotiate, to indicate that it is willing to consider change by lifting one of your index fingers. When one of your index fingers rises, thank it for its willingness to consider change and also for trying to help you cope with a situation. Respectfully remind it, however, that the way it is trying to help you, by making you tense, has become the problem. The tension is too great and, because of it, you are less able to tackle the situation.

Then access that part of the mind which we shall call the creative part of the mind. The part of the mind which weighs up the pro's and con's of everything you do. Ask it when it is listening and wanting to help with alternatives to raise the other index finger. When your other finger rises thank it for its willingness to help with alternative behaviours.

Now ask those two parts to get together in you unconscious mind to discuss and debate ways and means that will help you tackle the situation without making you tense. Let them be consultants for you, finding a few ways to help you cope with situations which would normally make you tense, without making you tense. Ask them, when they have found four or five ways to cope with the situations, without making you tense, to lift both your index fingers and bring them together, as a token of agreement. At this stage, because the negotiation has been going on in your unconscious mind you will not necessarily be aware of how they are going to help you. You should however find you have more options than being tense. Open your eyes and try some options. If the alternatives don't work repeat the exercise until they do.

Glossary

NEUROTIC BEHAVIOUR:—behaviour which generally leads to an increase of a problem and a move away from homeostasis.

HOMEOSTASIS:—a balanced, comfortable position in life.

HYPNOSIS:—a state of mind where there is a marked narrowing in the field of concentration with a corresponding increase in attention within that field.

HYPNOTIZABILITY:—the degree to which we are able to experience the state of hypnosis. This can be different and unique for each person, and not generally alterable. One method of measuring hypnotizability is Spiegel's Hypnotic Induction Profile, (see Spiegel's Trance and Treatment).

AUTO-HYPNOSIS:—hypnosis of self, by self.

BLAME GAME:—a game we all play, when we blame others or other things for how we feel. Feelings are personal experiences created by ourselves, for which we alone are responsible. If we blame others or other things then to get out of a feeling, others or other things are going to have to change. As this is unlikely to happen we are stuck and trapped in the feeling, if we play the blame game.

NEUROTIC NEEDS:—unsatisfied needs from the past projecting onto the present making us seek unreal satisfaction of those needs which are totally out of step with the present situation.

COSMIC CONSCIOUSNESS:—learned in the womb from having a dual consciousness of our selves and of being a part of mother at the same time. Like being a pebble on the beach and being the beach at the same time.

GLOSSARY

NEGATIVE IMPRINTING:—a once-and-for-all and one-off learning process due to an extremely negative experience.

PAVLOVIAN CONDITIONING:—a learning process which entails being subjected to repeated stimuli of the same nature until we learn to respond unconsciously.

OPERANT CONDITIONING:—a learning process which is nearly always goal-related where the behaviour earns a reward which may be positive or negative.

PRIMAL TRAUMA:—a term used by Arthur Janov in his books 'The Prima Scream. The Primal Revolution. The Anatomy of Mental Illness. The Feeling Child. Primal Man The New Consciousness. The Prisoner of Pain.' These traumas are not fully felt by the person experiencing them. The unfelt feeling being suppressed into the system (body or mind) remaining there and threatening to be felt for ever. The person with the primal pain having to suppress it for twenty-four hours a day, every day for the rest of their life.

FIRST LINE TRAUMA:—traumas experienced in the womb and at birth and for a few hours after birth giving rise to a particular set of behaviours. (See Arthur Janov's books for First, Second and Third Line traumas.)

SECOND LINE TRAUMA:—traumas experienced from a few hours after birth until about six years of age, generating another set of behaviours generally associated with an attempt to get attention due to the infant's inability to communicate, or the parents being unaware of their child's needs.

THIRD LINE TRAUMAS:—traumas occurring from about four years of age to the present day, generally caused between people (and the world) or each other giving rise to another set of different behaviours. There is an overlap of second and third line traumas depending on the child's needs at the time of the trauma. All these terms are described in full by Janov in his books.

PRIMAL ANCHOR:—a set of circumstances often remote from the behaviour but, which nevertheless, has attached to them, and promotes unconsciously a particular behaviour which may be positive or negative.

PRIMAL GATES:—the method by which a person holds back unfelt primal pain in his, or her, system.

PRIMAL THERAPY:—described by Arthur Janov in his books (see PRIMAL TRAUMA above).

REFRAMING:—a method of changing behaviour by reprogramming the 'bio-computer' we call our mind by offering it an alternative behaviour to solve a problem. It is hoped this new behaviour will lead to a more satisfactory solution and a state nearer to homeostasis. (See book Reframing by Richard Bandler and John Grinder.)

ABREAT-ABREACTION:—a reliving of an experience with a full expression of the emotions attached to that experience.

BONDING:—a necessary psychological function created very shortly after birth by eye to eye contact between baby and, hopefully, loving parent.

SPLIT SCREEN TECHNIQUE (SPIEGEL):—a technique for reprogramming the 'bio-computer' we call our mind described by Spiegel in Donald S. Connery's book THE INNER SOURCE, published by Holt, Rinehart and Winston, New York.

IDEO-MOTOR FINGER RESPONSE:—a technique consisting of wording questions to the unconscious mind so they can be answered 'yes' or 'no', to uncover dynamic processes in the unconscious mind. This technique was first described by David Cheek and Leslie LeCron in their book 'Clinical Hypnotherapy' published by Grune and Stratton 1968.

REACTIVE DEPRESSION:—a depression as a reaction to a disaster, family tragedy, or individual misfortune, which goes on long after normal grief, or sorrow, should have ended.

ANOREXIA NERVOSA:—the 'slimmers disease' which is often fatal.

REBIRTHING:—techniques of getting a person to relive their birth with the expression of feelings experienced at that time (birth). Using their adult knowledge to experience that time (birth) they can often make new decisions about the birth which, hopefully, will enable them to have alternative behaviours. (See chapter 7.)

GESTALT THERAPY:—a technique of psychotherapy described by Frederick Perls, Ralph Hefferline and Paul Goodman in their book 'Gestalt Therapy' published by Julian Press New York 1951

E.C.T.:—a technique of passing an electric shock through the brain, used as a treatment for depression.

ORGANIC BRAIN DISFUNCTION (O.B.D.):—work done by David McGlown and Peter Blyth in Chester showing that if the Tonic Neck Reflex, Unilateral reflex and Cross lateral reflexes are not present due to incorrect developmental learning, the person without these reflexes will exhibit a number of physical and psychological difficulties in later life.

RELATIVE ANALGESIA:—a technique using a mixture of Nitrous Oxide and Oxygen as a method of sedation and pain relief. Can be used to lower resistance in hypnosis, or to break through primal gates in primal therapy.

Bibliography

BLYTH, PETER—McGLOWN, DAVID:—two psychologists who were working together in Chester, England and are now working independently on various aspects of psychology and psychotherapy.

CHEEK, DAVID, M.D F.A.C.S., F.A.C.O.G.:—Diplomate, American Board of Obstetrics and Gynaecology; Past President, American Society of Clinical Hypnosis. CoAuthor 'Clinical Hypnotherapy' Grune and Stratton New York.

DELECATO and DOLMAN:—Directors of the Institute of Human Potential in Philadelphia.

DUNCAN, SHEILA:—'Company of wolves' Sunday Times, 11 November 1984. Sheila Duncan talks to Jinnie Jefferies about rape therapy for violent prisoners.

ELMAN, DAVE:—Author 'Findings in Hypnosis' published Pauline R. Elman 1964. Ref. (2) page 5.

FERENCZI, SANDOR:—Ferenczi's reasoning was to the effect that neurotics are people who have never been properly loved and accepted as children by their real parents. What disturbed people most need is a therapist who, as substitute parent, will let them relive their childhood experiences in a completely warm, loving, permissive atmosphere. These reasonings were described by Ferenczi in 1927.

FREUD, SIGMUND:—the pioneer of psychoanalytic theory and practice. Freud claimed that birth was our first trauma and the origin of all anxieties at the root of later psychological problems. 'The Basic Writings of Sigmund Freud' (translated by A. A. Brill) New York: Modern Library, 1938.

GRAHAM, GEOFFREY:—Author of this book. See Curriculum Vitae.

BIBLIOGRAPHY

GROF, STANISLAV:—Author of 'Realms of the Human Unconscious' published by Dutton 1976, and 'L.S.D. Psychotherapy.' published by Hunter House, 1980.

HOLMES and RAHE:—working for the United States Navy responsible for the scale of STRESS OF ADJUSTING TO CHANGE.

JANOV, ARTHUR:—Author of 'The Primal Scream', 'The Primal Revolution', 'The Anatomy of Mental Illness', 'The Feeling Child', 'Primal Man', 'Prisoner of Pain'.

LAKE, FRANK:— Author of 'Clinical Theology' 1976, and 'Tight Corners in Pastoral Counselling' 1981. Both published by Dartman, Longman and Todd.

LANGA, HARRY:—Author 'Relative Analgesia in Dental Practice' published W. B. Saunders Company, 1976.

LEBOYER, FREDERIC:—French Obstetrician Gynaecologist with a film on Natural Childbirth.

LOWEN ALEXANDER:—Author 'Bioenergetics' published Coward. MC Cann and Geoghegan. inc. New York, 1975.

PAVLOV:—a distinguished Russian physiologist developed the conditioned Reflex theory of learning.

RANK, OTTO:—Author of 'The Trauma of Birth'.

REICH, WILHELM:—Author of 'Character Analysis'. Vision Press Ltd. 1950

SPIEGEL, HERBERT:—Author of 'Trance and Treatment', Basic Books, New York. 1978. Ref. (1) and (3) page 5.

TILLEARD-COLE, RICHARD R.,:—Author 'The Fundamentals of Psychological medicine'. Medical and Technical Publishing Co. Ltd. 1975. Director of the Oxford Institute of Psychiatry, Oxford.

To re-order for a friend or patient by mail order send to—

REAL OPTIONS PRESS, Dunsopp House, Lucy Street, Blaydon upon Tyne. NE21 5PU. U.K.

------- Cut here

Please send...... copies of 'How To Become The Parent You Never Had' to

Name ....

Address ....

....

....

....

Post Code ....

I enclose £6.95 + £1.05 (post and package) for each book U.K. market or $10 + $6 (post and package) for U.S.A. market.

------- Cut here

Book by the same author available by 1st April 1987

'IT'S A BIT OF A MOUTHFUL'

With self help exercises for Obesity, Smoking, Alcoholism, Oral Sex, Anorexia Nervosa, Nail Biting, Thumb Sucking, Dental Phobia and other Dental Problems.

Please send...... copies of IT'S A BIT OF A MOUTHFUL to

Name ....

Address ....

....

....

....

Post Code ....

I enclose £6.95 + £1.05 (post and package) for each book U.K. market or $10 + $6 (post and package) for U.S.A. market.

Please send the completed order to Real Options Press, Dunsopp House, Lucy Street, Blaydon upon Tyne. NE21 5PU. U.K.
Please print Name and Address clearly.

To re-order for a friend or patient by mail order send to—

REAL OPTIONS PRESS, Dunsopp House, Lucy Street, Blaydon upon Tyne. NE21 5PU. U.K.

-- Cut here

Please send...... copies of 'How To Become The Parent You Never Had' to

Name ....

Address ....

....

....

....

Post Code.............................

I enclose £6.95 + £1.05 (post and package) for each book U.K. market or $10 + $6 (post and package) for U.S.A. market.

-- Cut here

Book by the same author available by 1st April 1987

'IT'S A BIT OF A MOUTHFUL'

With self help exercises for Obesity, Smoking, Alcoholism, Oral Sex, Anorexia Nervosa, Nail Biting, Thumb Sucking, Dental Phobia and other Dental Problems.

Please send...... copies of IT'S A BIT OF A MOUTHFUL to

Name ....

Address ....

....

....

....

Post Code.............................

I enclose £6.95 + £1.05 (post and package) for each book U.K. market or $10 + $6 (post and package) for U.S.A. market.

Please send the completed order to Real Options Press, Dunsopp House, Lucy Street, Blaydon upon Tyne. NE21 5PU. U.K.
Please print Name and Address clearly.